MICROCOMPUTERS IN HEALTH CARE MANAGEMENT

William W. Christensen
Administrative Associate

Eugene I. Stearns
Associate Administrator

Main Hospital and W.K. Kellogg Eye Center
University of Michigan Hospitals

AN ASPEN PUBLICATION®
Aspen Publishers, Inc.
Rockville, Maryland
Royal Tunbridge Wells
1984

Library of Congress Cataloging in Publication Data

Christensen, William W.
Microcomputers in health care management.

"An Aspen publication."
Includes index.
1. Health facilities — Administration — Data processing.
2. Microcomputers. I. Stearns, Eugene I. II. Title.
[DNLM: 1. Computers. 2. Health Services — organization & administration. W 26.5 C554m]
RA971.6.C47 1984 362.1'068 84-6491
ISBN: 0-89443-596-5

Publisher: John R. Marozsan
Associate Publisher: Jack W. Knowles, Jr.
Editor-in-Chief: Michael Brown
Executive Managing Editor: Margot G. Raphael
Managing Editor: M. Eileen Higgins
Editorial Services: Ruth Bloom
Printing and Manufacturing: Debbie Collins

Library of Congress Catalog Card Number: 84-6491
ISBN: 0-89443-596-5

Printed in the United States of America

3 4 5

To

John, Barbery, and Bobbie Christensen

and

Leslie, David, Randy, and Joey Stearns

Table of Contents

Preface

Having accepted the premise that microcomputers are becoming a part of the everyday life of hospitals and other health care organizations, we have written this book for health care managers who work at every level of management. Administrators will benefit by gaining insight into the value and limitations of microcomputers specifically and of computing in general. Many administrators who are not now computer "literate" (i.e., who have little knowledge of the nature, value, or internal workings of computers) will achieve a reasonable degree of computer literacy having read this book. Managers and first line supervisors will recognize that they can learn to solve often complex problems by applying a powerful but relatively inexpensive technology in their day-to-day work.

It is our intention to provide a balanced examination of the benefits and advantages as well as the limits and pitfalls of microcomputing in the health care setting.

Microcomputers in Health Care Management is also intended to be readable. Whatever technical language it contains is defined and explained in the second chapter, "State of the Art." Chapter 2 also provides sufficient background and technical information so the reader can understand and use the rest of the material presented.

Chapter 1 begins with a brief historical perspective on the advent of mainframe computing and traces the development of large computers and minicomputers to the present proliferation of microcomputers for business and other uses. The relative costs of using these different sizes of computers are discussed, as are the potential benefits and difficulties involved in using both large and small computers.

The basic concepts, terms, and functions used throughout the book are introduced in Chapter 2. A detailed comparison of the existing types and capabilities of microcomputing equipment is given as well.

Chapter 3 explores the use of microcomputers in the hospital environment. The following subjects are covered:

- orchestrating microcomputer program development
- using strategies to introduce the microcomputer to an office
- understanding and dealing with the differences between microcomputers and mainframes
- identifying and avoiding the pitfalls of microcomputer development
- instituting controls

In Chapter 4, the use of spreadsheet programs is described. The general idea of an "electronic spreadsheet" is explained and an exploration of specific functions of spreadsheet programs is provided. Almost 50 examples of electronic spreadsheet models, many relating to specific departments, are given as a means of showing the power of spreadsheet programs. These models are also meant to provide a springboard from which readers can develop their own imaginative uses.

Because inexpensive word processing "packages" are available for many micros (some vendors even provide word processing as part of special purchase agreements) the micro can be put to productive use immediately, if desired, even while you are becoming familiar with the equipment. Chapter 5 considers word processing on a microcomputer, including the following points:

- advantages and disadvantages
- examples of word processing programs used on selected micros
- dedicated word processing systems

Chapter 6 deals with data base management on a microcomputer. One of the more useful applications related to data base management is the tracking system. The general benefits of a computerized tracking system (both from a personal as well as an institutional point of view) are presented, as are the limitations of using micros for such tasks. Several software packages are described in order to give the potential user a framework for software purchasing or development decisions. The use of data base management programs is covered in easy to understand language. Also included is a program developed by the authors for project tracking.

Microcomputer graphics programs are described and explained in Chapter 7. Applications for a number of different departments are included, illustrating the range of microcomputer-based graphics.

Finally, three appendixes are included. Appendix A contains a glossary of terms used throughout the book. Appendix B is a guide for designing, writing, and implementing a microcomputer program from scratch. While not every manager may have an interest in doing programming, understanding how it is done is still important. How else is the manager to know if the programmer being hired has the required skills? Knowledge of systems and programming fundamentals will help the manager communicate more effectively with those who are writing the actual programs. Managers need this insight into the workings, capabilities, and limitations of present microcomputer systems. They also need to have some sense of the expected future developments in the field.

In order to write an effective program, it is necessary to determine the size of your task. How to accomplish this is explained in Appendix C. To obtain the greatest benefit from this section, Appendix B should be read first. Appendix C will help the reader determine the best manner in which to proceed in solving a problem using microcomputer assistance. The reader is also advised to read Chapter 2 before proceeding, because definitions of the terms and concepts used are given there.

Please note that all computer models, company names, and programs mentioned in this book are trademarks. The reader is urged to secure literature and appropriate dealer assistance in exploring microcomputer applications to his or her particular health care management needs.

Acknowledgments

The authors would like to take this opportunity to acknowledge the assistance of the many individuals who helped us produce this book. We thank Leslie Stearns for her patience and understanding during a rather prolonged writing and production process. We would particularly like to thank Carl Zang, Coordinator, Financial Reporting, at the University of Michigan Hospitals for his thoughtful comments and contributions related to using spreadsheet and graphics software, as well as Randy Wright of the Complete Computer Center in Ann Arbor for his perspective on the microcomputer field. We would also like to thank Joseph M. Spallina, Senior Consultant, Chi Systems, Inc.

We would like to thank the following individuals at the University of Michigan Hospitals in Ann Arbor for their comments related to their areas of expertise: Norma Grills (Director, Dietetics), Judy Asiala (Assistant Director, Medical Records), Jean Robinson (Director, Social Work), Brian Moore (Material Management), and Linda Vader, R.N. (Head Nurse, Kellogg Eye Center).

We would like to express our appreciation to the editorial staff of Aspen Systems for their encouragement and forbearance over the long process of book production, particularly Mike Brown, Sandy Cannon, and Ruth Bloom.

Chapter 1

Introduction

The explosion of miniaturized technology that occurred in the last half of the 1970s produced an almost mind-boggling array of microcomputers that are available at costs ranging downward from $25,000 to less than $100. As a result, microcomputers have become household items. Most schools now use them both as instructional aids in the "Three R's" and as the basis for the development of computer literacy.

Today, most students are beginning to learn about computer programming no later than in junior high school. Many have encountered computers in elementary school and some even in the primary grades. The schools perceive the value of and need for computer literacy and have responded with enthusiasm.

In the near future, working adults who have been educated by these schools will have an expertise not now possessed by many managers and administrators. This growing cadre of people who are computer "literate," that is, who understand what computers do and how they do it, will become a major competitive force in the labor market. They will be in a position to provide the institutions and businesses where they are employed with a set of tools that are now understood and possessed by only a few. Moreover, in the not-too-distant future, graduates entering the management ranks will have expectations different from those held by many of today's managers when they entered the field. Job applicants who encounter an office setting that offers few, if any, types of sophisticated computer or word processing equipment might be likened to those in the 1960s who found offices without electric typewriters.

Attracting the best, most qualified managers will undoubtedly require a display of computing sophistication not now found in most hospitals or other health care facilities. To provide such a work setting and gain the benefits of new technologies, administrators must become better informed about possibilities and opportunities. They must be aware of the capabilities and limitations of this technology.

In some instances, a department may desire or need to develop specific information-handling tools that are not commercially available and that are not likely to be developed because of their limited applicability. Under these circumstances, the task of attracting persons who possess microcomputer expertise should not be very difficult. Many people are available who, while perhaps not formally trained in computer technology, nevertheless, through their schoolwork, previous jobs, or the presence of a microcomputer in their homes have come to possess sufficient expertise to do simple programming at a very satisfactory level. Formally trained computer programmers and system analysts are not as easy to find, and usually would be expected to command higher salaries.

In some cases, the size of tasks to be supported by a microcomputer is such that formally trained programmers are needed. If so, there are several things users can do to attract them. One is to assure them that adequate hardware has been allocated. Another is to provide an environment and enough time for creative work. Prospective programming employees should understand that working in a more specialized management situation is likely to result in greater freedom and flexibility for them.

This book is not directed at people who are interested in developing large systems that require significant personnel support. The aim, rather, is to assist managers in developing tools that will enable them to better cope with the daily pressures of work and the planning and evaluation of work processes and outcomes. These are typically problem-solving tools that allow managers to use information about their operations.

USING INFORMATION

The information needed to solve problems is often stored in large computers, but much of the time it may be difficult to retrieve in a desired form or format. Often data can be transferred from computerized reports for reentry into a microcomputer and then processed efficiently to produce "new" information. This is accomplished by analyzing the data differently, such as by sorting differently, performing different mathematical calculations, or making new comparisons. For example, the central computer may produce the following paper report:

	Budget	Expense	Variance	Pct.
Payroll	10000	9000	1000	10
Commodities	8000	6000	2000	25
Total	18000	15000	3000	16.6

That is rather simple and straightforward. Now, assume you also have another report, this one related to patient days or patient diagnosis grouping. (These reports could have been produced by a computer but there is no reason they have to be; they could have been manually produced as well.) A patient day report might look like this:

Patient Day Report

	December	YTD	Dec. Budget	YTD Budget
Unit A	658	7396	600	7200
Unit B	400	4650	390	4630
Total	1058	12046	990	11830

If you were interested in knowing the payroll or commodities costs per patient day, a number of calculations would be required. A simple "spreadsheet" program could be constructed that would allow you to enter data from each report and "massage" it in ways that would produce the information you are after. Your new information might look like this:

Cost Per Patient Day

	Patient Days		Expenses		Cost/Patient Day	
	Budget	Act.	Budget	Act.	Budget	Act.
Payroll	990	1058	10000	9000	10.10	8.51
Commodity	990	1058	8000	6000	8.08	5.67
Total	990	1058	18000	15000	18.18	14.18

Obviously, this is a very simple example using a small amount of data. Performing a small number of calculations would not cause one to think about turning to a microcomputer. But imagine having to perform a number of such calculations, say filling 25 or 50 lines with numbers arrayed over eight or ten columns. Then the problem would look more like that in Exhibit 1-1.

Each figure in this example is calculated by dividing the number by each item used in a given month by the patient day figure for that month. The effort required to manually perform the repeated calculations needed to produce this information is not only costly and time consuming but frustrating for people whose job does not typically involve manipulating numbers.

Moreover, the cost of repetitive manipulations of data is much lower using microcomputers than electronic calculators, and the additional cost of data entry can be surprisingly low because the data may have been put into summary form by the mainframe computer or some other method.

Allowing managers to experiment with new techniques can produce outstanding results. When the "specialist" in the office is made to feel comfortable and free, the rewards will be considerable and far reaching.

Exhibit 1-1 Linen Usage per Patient Day

LINEN USAGE FOR FISCAL 1982			COST	JULY	AUG	SEPT	OCT	NOV	DEC	TOTAL	JAN	FEB	MAR	APRL	MAY	JUNE	TOTAL
LINEN BAGS	9010105	EACH	0.23	51	46	46	41	62	39	285	46	48	46	51	48	55	580
BATHROBES	9010257	EACH	0.22	10	17	17	11	14	9	77	12	10	26	25	10	10	184
BATH BLANKETS	9010658	EACH	0.29	58	46	58	55	81	52	351	73	88	52	64	52	64	722
CLEANING CLOTHS		LB.	0.23	7	2	5	5	0	7	25	5	0	5	2	2	2	44
PATIENT GOWNS	9012059	EACH	0.28	35	48	43	32	48	38	244	29	35	28	28	20	28	398
PAJAMA TOPS	9012503	EACH	0.11	38	43	41	31	38	25	216	57	34	79	56	23	30	530
PAJAMA BOTTOMS	9012606	EACH	0.11	38	47	40	31	37	21	213	40	34	68	56	23	30	486
PILLOW CASES	9012953	EACH	0.07	39	45	50	34	56	34	258	45	48	46	50	36	49	526
LARGE SHEETS	9013209	EACH	0.34	238	272	272	204	306	204	1496	272	290	262	299	218	306	3128
BED SPREADS	9014706	EACH	0.56	76	76	81	70	104	62	468	50	84	73	76	53	84	865
SOCKS	9014408	EACH	0.02	4	4	4	4	4	2	22	6	3	10	7	2	4	56
BATH TOWELS	9014901	EACH	0.11	105	99	116	94	121	88	622	110	99	132	143	83	132	1353
WASH CLOTHS	9015450	EACH	0.01	10	10	11	9	11	8	59	11	18	11	13	8	12	125
	TOTALS			708	754	783	619	881	588	4334	755	790	837	870	577	805	8996

ENTERING THE WORLD OF THE MICROCOMPUTER

At least as important, if not more important than attracting the specialist with computer expertise, is the way management and supervisory staff are acclimated to the microcomputer. In the past, microcomputers were called toys, often by the promoters of large computers who sometimes have disdain for them. However, with its vast array of potentials and capabilities, the microcomputer may be the single most important reason for the current "demystification" of the world of computers. Some people have expressed the opinion that the purveyors of the "computer myth" have for years kept a clever secret about how computers work—what better way to maintain a monopoly on computer expertise (not to mention jobs)? But the situation is changing rapidly. As microcomputers are showing up in hundreds of thousands of households, as "personal computers," and in like numbers of businesses, both large and small, as "professional computers," the immediate access to them by workers, parents, and students increases dramatically. Today, there are scores of magazines devoted to personal computing, hundreds of training manuals, educational programs, and innumerable books. Computer stores have sprouted and are thriving all over the country.

In this milieu, health care administrators and managers may feel anxious or awkward. Encouragement to use microcomputers, rather than misunderstand and fear them, can do much to alleviate the situation. Even the mere availability of a microcomputer or terminal prompts use by managers. This surely has something to do with the desire to save time and effort, to have as much good information as possible, and to deal with the fear of not being competitive.

The following is a simple strategy for encouraging managers to use the microcomputer:

1. Set up a micro in a quiet place.
2. Enter a video game people can play (make sure it has educational value).
3. In a day or two, replace the game with information about how people can learn to use the computer.
4. Place instructional materials and several canned programs nearby—word processing programs provide a familiar starting point.
5. Make some "expertise" available—either an employee to serve as instructor and guide, a minicourse (many computer stores offer them), or whatever assistance is available from your own institution's information center, if it has one

6. Set up a control person to monitor use—you will need this because within a short time the computer will be busy and fully subscribed.
7. Add micros—you will probably need them. They are inexpensive.

What the institution will end up with is a group of managers and administrators who think about problem solving somewhat differently, who will for the most part be better informed, and who will keep others better informed.

ACQUIRING THE MICROCOMPUTER

Acquiring a microcomputer for specialized intradepartmental use, such as for word processing or spreadsheet programs, should not entail a great deal of discussion with the data processing department, except insofar as technical advice may be sought or rendered. The implementation of a microcomputer for relatively straightforward uses such as these is not difficult to accomplish. On the other hand, the development of larger systems involving linkages, security, and communication with a "host" computer or other micros will demand thoughtful institutional planning at a relatively high level. The trick is to be able to discriminate so as to avoid bogging down the small departmental application in needless red tape while preserving the necessary degree of managerial rigor required for developing larger systems. A method for justifying microcomputer implementation is discussed in Chapter 3.

Because it might be difficult to acquire micros in some settings, the following guidelines may be helpful for overcoming obstacles and avoiding pitfalls.

Education

One of the major obstacles to acquiring microcomputer capabilities in a large organization like a hospital is lack of knowledge about microcomputers at the higher policy-making levels. This does not necessarily reflect built-in bias or prejudice, but simply a lack of understanding that often leads to management inertia. A full-scale attack on ignorance is needed to publicize the potential benefits of microcomputing. Drive home the features of cost effectiveness, speed of turnaround, graphics capabilities, convenience, user friendliness, portability, and the large number of software programs on the market. If you have the authority, purchase a reasonable size system, one that will benefit your operation, and use the results you attain to make your point. (If you are the chief executive officer, educate the Board.)

Cooperation

For years hospitals and other health care organizations of all sizes have been in the continuous process of acquiring and using large computer system support (whether through inhouse facilities, contract services, or time sharing). The result may be that in some installations there is a perceived need to protect one's "turf." One can understand the reluctance of a data processing manager to consider a large number of autonomous or integrated small computer systems if a large financial commitment has been made to developing a centralized computer service. However, most data processing managers do understand the value of all types of computer capability and are more than willing to discuss ways of accommodating smaller machines within the total framework of health care computing.

Health care managers should discuss and objectively clarify the functional differences, roles, advantages, and disadvantages of micro and mainframe computers with their data processing or information system managers. For example, the following lists might be mutually agreed upon:

Advantages of Microcomputers

- single function by a single operator at a time
- intradepartmental scope
- high capability for "what if" statistics that are department or unit specific
- low volume data entry and retention requirements
- applications that are controlled by the department manager for the department's specific information needs
- stand-alone applications that would not otherwise be accomplished on the mainframe computer
- applications that provide a number of different scenarios based on the same data and requiring many computer "runs"

Advantages of Mainframe Computers

- multiple simultaneous functions by multiple users
- interdepartmentally integrated scope
- high volume data entry and retention requirements

- applications that are controlled by top management for meeting the overall information needs of the organization

Especially important is an understanding of the wide range of specific applications that can and should be performed on a microcomputer rather than on a large mainframe computer. These include:

- using the micro as an inexpensive but powerful word processing machine
- using the micro to test and debug mainframe program algorithms and overall system approaches
- allowing the micro to perform stand-alone computer tasks that should not (or would not) otherwise be accomplished on a large computer
- utilizing the micro for small-scale data base management
- assigning to the micro repetitive tasks that do not warrant major programming efforts on a mainframe computer (e.g., multiple scenarios on an electronic spreadsheet)

The central computer management hierarchy should be engaged in frank discussions about the need for, value, limitations, and expectations of microcomputers. Computer managers are usually open to new technologies (it's one of the reasons they are in the field). On those rare occasions when the computer manager attempts to block a legitimate effort, a serious person will seek to determine the cause. Sometimes, the thinking is sound. There may be many reasons to control the spread and use of microcomputers; these should be discussed openly. If, on the other hand, obstacles are being thrown up solely because of anxiety or turf guarding, continued effort is needed in order to educate those at higher levels. Managers must be persistent in their attempts to acquire the tools they can legitimately use to advantage for their institutions.

Perspective

While attempting to overcome any obstacles to microcomputer acquisition, it is essential to continue to work at what should be considered the main task at hand, choosing from among the available hardware and software that will suit your needs and committing these resources to the goals of your department and institution. How to do this will be explained in the chapters that follow.

Chapter 2

State of the Art

In this chapter, the nature of microcomputing will be explored by presenting both the hardware and software advances that make these small systems possible. It is essential that the beginner spend the time necessary to become familiar with the concepts and terms introduced in this chapter; the computer expert will also find items of value.

Two basic terms that should be introduced immediately are hardware and software. Hardware is the actual physical aspect of the computer: the keys on the keyboard, the chips in the memory, and so on. Software is the set of instructions that tells the computer what to do; this software is typically (in the case of micros) stored on floppy disks or hard disk devices until it is needed.

HARDWARE

When first introduced, computers were single creations, each one more of a research prototype than a multipurpose machine. The intentions of the designers were twofold: to explore the practical and technical implications of the works of such mathematicians as Von Neumann and Turing and to satisfy the needs of their sponsors.

These machines were, in fact, built for a single purpose; the "program," or function, of the machine was physically present in the design of the electrical circuitry. To change the "program" the entire machine had to be taken apart and rebuilt. Programming took many weeks of painstaking engineering effort.

As the design of computers progressed, the modern conception of the computer as a multipurpose device that would readily accept new sets of instructions came into being. The computer evolved into a universal, practical tool that consists of the following logical units:

1. Central processing unit, including the control unit and arithmetic and logical unit
2. Memory
3. Input unit
4. Output unit

In the following sections, the logical units of a computer will be explored, with particular emphasis on the hardware used with microcomputers. The information applies to both mini and mainframe computers, with the exception of hardware specifications.

The Central Processing Unit

The central processing unit (also called the processor or the CPU) includes two logical units, the control unit and the arithmetic and logical unit. The control unit regulates the entire computer system and ensures that program statements, commands, and data are properly routed throughout the system. The arithmetic and logical unit performs all the mathematical tasks assigned (e.g., addition and subtraction, sine and cosine, square roots and squares), as well as the necessary actions related to logic statements within programs (e.g., statements like IF X = 10, THEN PRINT "10").

The microcomputer industry is the direct beneficiary of the technology called Large Scale Integration (or LSI). This technology is what puts the "micro" into microprocessor, by allowing the replacement of thousands of distinct physical units of the computers of the 1950s and 1960s with a single chip. Rather than wire together many discrete pieces to form the logic and capacity of the computer, we can now etch the gates and cells that replace them into the surface of tiny crystals. Often, the CPU and part of the memory are placed on a single chip; this technology dates from the mid 1970s.

Memory

The memory used by the computer takes several different forms, the two major divisions being based on the hardware involved.

Main Memory

The first, called "main memory," is the area to which the computer has the fastest access. Today, most main memory units for microcomputers are LSI integrated circuits (ICs); these are the tiny "chips" that form the heart of the modern computer. If you look inside a micro, a number of small black boxes with tiny pins sticking out of the bottom can be seen arranged in neat rows; these plastic boxes each contain a small (roughly ⅛ inch square) chip that forms the actual IC.

The most common forms of internal memory are random access memory (RAM) and read only memory (ROM). The RAM space is the area into which the program statements and data are entered and worked on. It is called random access because the computer can get to any part of it at once, without having to look through each of the cells preceding the desired location. It may be useful to compare a tape recording of a concert consisting of, say, 20 songs with a record album containing the same songs. If you want to listen to (or "access") the seventh song on the tape recording, you must go through the songs preceding it; however, to reach the same song on the record, you can skip directly to the song you want. The record and record player thus constitute a random access storage system.

The RAM in a computer contains no information when you turn the machine on; it forms the major workspace of the machine. Transfer from cell to cell occurs at the fastest rate available to the user. This is important because all of the operations performed by the computer consist of transfers of information from one cell to another. The faster this transfer takes place, the sooner the computer will complete its work.

The ROM memory is very similar, except that you can only read its contents; the data written on it are permanent and cannot be written over. It is a form of permanent storage, whereas the RAM space is like a scratchpad that can be written on, erased, and written on again.

One of the most important limitations on the usefulness of microcomputers is the size of the RAM space available; the amount of RAM that can be used is determined by the CPU chosen for that particular computer. Most micros are limited to a range of from 64,000 to 512,000 bytes (that is, storage "cells") of this kind of space.

In addition to being limited in size, another problem with RAM memory is that it is volatile; that is, when the power to the computer is turned off, whatever is stored in it is lost. To make up for these limitations, a second kind of memory is needed, which is more permanent and not limited in size by the CPU; this is referred to as the mass memory.

Mass Memory

A number of different hardware devices are used to provide mass memory to microcomputers. The following major types can be distinguished:

1. Tape recorder
2. Floppy disk drive

3. Hard disk drive
4. Solid state (IC) devices

Tape Recorder. Most microcomputers can use a standard tape recorder to store data and programs. This technology is not greatly developed, however, because it is not a very satisfactory storage method for most users. Because tape recorders are not random access devices, finding what you want on the tape can be a slow process (as you know if you've ever gone hunting for a tape of your favorite song). Also, the rate of data transfer between the recorder and the computer is very slow (on the order of 30 characters per second). However, tape recordings of data and programs are utilized by a significant number of users as a means of "backup" storage. Tapes are inexpensive and accept a large amount of data. Tape recorders are sometimes the only available storage medium for low-cost computers, again because of the modest price of tape recorders.

Floppy Disk Drive. The floppy disk drive represents a significant advance over the tape recorder as a means of storage in several respects. First, it is a random access device, like a record player. In fact, the floppy disk itself consists of a flexible plastic record inside a special envelope. The disk is spun at a high speed and read from and written upon by a head sitting very close to the surface of the record. The disk itself is covered with magnetically sensitive particles (just like a recording tape). When recording information on the disk, the head causes magnetic patterns in these particles to appear, which can then be interpreted later. As with a record player, disks can be removed and stored when the disk has been filled with information.

Floppy disks were originally designed for minicomputers; the size of the first floppies was 8 inches. The microcomputer industry developed its own version, a 5¼ inch floppy disk. Because the unit is smaller and typically stores information in a less dense format, the 5¼ inch floppy disk drives could be manufactured more cheaply. Most microcomputer floppy disks can store from 100,000 to 400,000 bytes of information.

These devices also have a much higher data transfer rate because the disk is spinning very rapidly, on the order of 400 rpm. Compare the speed at which the tape in a tape recorder moves past the recording head with the rate at which the surface of the floppy disk is moving past its recording head.

The floppy disk system also includes a special section reserved for a catalog of all files stored on the disk as well as a program that allows the computer to make easy use of this catalog. Thus, if you wish to get the file labeled "September Payroll," you merely type the access command

and the filename, in the case of the Apple II, "LOAD SEPTEMBER PAYROLL." The computer then does the rest.

Hard Disk Drive. The hard disk drive is almost identical to the floppy disk drive; in fact, floppy disks were developed from hard disks. The major difference is that the hard disk system is sealed; the disks are (typically) not removable. This allows the disk to spin faster and enables the head to float closer to the surface of the disk, thus speeding up the process of reading data from the disk.

Also, the hard disk stores more data per disk; typically from 5 to 20 million bytes (5 to 20 Megabytes) per disk. This makes up for the fact that you cannot change disks when you fill one up (in the case of most hard disk drive units).

For a number of years, the distinction between floppy disks and hard disks was clearly drawn. However, this line has blurred considerably in recent years. For example, there are now available, at a higher cost, hard disk drives that have removable hard disk units; these units combine the best of floppies and hard disks. On the other end of the spectrum, hard disks are now being made that store information in a very dense format, one that requires special cartridges and closer tolerances in the drive mechanism; these systems closely approach the data density of hard disks. These 3½ inch micro floppies are considered by many to be the new industry standard—one that will replace the 5¼ inch floppy disk.

In addition, hard disks are becoming available in smaller sizes at a cheaper price; 8 inch and 5¼ inch sizes have been available for some time but hard disks as small as 3½ inches are now being manufactured.

Solid State Devices. The final mass storage technology to be considered is the solid state device. Such devices are also called disk drive emulators, because they respond to queries from the computer exactly as a disk drive does. The difference is that the data are stored on ICs within the device, exactly as in the main computer. Solid state devices are available as separate units that look like disk drives from the outside; they are also available as cards that plug into the main body of the computer itself.

These devices have been made possible by the rapidly diminishing cost of integrated circuits. In January of 1977, the retail cost of 16,000 bytes of RAM memory (chips only) was approximately $650; by 1982, a complete 130,000 byte RAM storage device could be purchased for about the same price.

In the coming years, the trend in microcomputers will almost certainly move toward greater use of solid state devices rather than mechanical devices. The history of computing has demonstrated a uniform trend away from moving parts and toward solid state. A device with no moving parts can typically be made more cheaply, with fewer defects, lower power consumption, and a smaller chance of failure. The dramatic drop in the price of RAM chips is typical of the shrinking cost of solid state technology.

The Input Unit

Input unit is a general term for the device that allows instructions and data to be entered into the machine. In the case of a microcomputer this is the keyboard.

The Keyboara

There is wide variation in keyboards in the microcomputer industry. Some look almost exactly like the keyboard of a typical electric typewriter (e.g., the Apple II); some keyboards are very complex and technical in appearance. All micro keyboards follow the usual QWERTY convention for alphabetic characters but the resemblance stops there.

Many micro keyboards include a keypad (for numeric data entry) and keys to control the movement of the cursor on the screen of the system. Because the keyboard is the part of the computer that you spend the most time with, it is important to look at it with the following criteria in mind:

1. Is it too threatening for what you need it to do? If you are doing primarily word processing, you may not require a large 90+ key keyboard.
2. Does it feel comfortable? Do you prefer sculpted rows, keys that depress and contact in a particular way?
3. Are you used to a certain arrangement of the nonalphabetic keys?

The user typically must make some sort of tradeoff; the keyboard is not the most important part of the machine. Most micro manufacturers are very sensitive to the needs of users; the model you choose should fit your needs in as many categories as possible.

It should also be noted that there are a number of manufacturers providing separate numeric keypads for those machines that do not have built-in ones. This can be particularly helpful if you are using your machine primarily for accounting.

The Joystick

Another class of input devices allows the user to "point" to something on the screen. Most people are familiar with the joystick controls present on many computer game machines, both in arcades and in small home computers. The joystick is a rod attached to sensors placed in an upright position; the position corresponds to a point on the computer screen. Moving the stick out of the perpendicular causes the sensors to record a new position for the spot based on the new position of the rod. Moving the rod tip to the lower right causes the spot on the screen to move to the lower right, and so on. Alternatives can be chosen from a list by moving the spot with the joystick until it corresponds with the alternative desired; pushing a button tells the computer that you have made your choice.

The Mouse

Another mechanism used for this purpose is the mouse. The mouse is a small box that has a trackball in the bottom that rolls along when the mouse is pushed along a surface. The motion of the ball is translated into motion of a spot on the screen. The mouse has a button that may be pushed when a choice has been completed. This particular device is very popular with users who do not like the keyboard. For this reason, some people believe the mouse may make microcomputers more accessible to higher level executives. (Studies have shown that many top-level executives dislike the idea of using computers because they believe the typing involved lowers their status. If much of a user's interaction with the machine takes place through some sort of pointing device, this problem may be alleviated.)

Light Pen

The light pen is another input device that is available with microcomputers that is used to point physically to a portion of the screen. Typically, the program is set up with a number of alternatives, each marked with a special character that is recognized by the light pen, and its associated software. By placing the light pen on the special character (pressing the pen against the screen), an alternative may be chosen.

Touch Sensitive Screen

The final input device to be considered here is the touch sensitive screen. In this case, the user may select from alternatives by physically using a finger to point to and press a section of the screen corresponding to the choice to be made.

The Output Unit

The output unit may be any of several devices, including mass storage devices, printers, monitors, and telecommunications. As we have already looked at the mass storage devices, let us examine the other devices available with microcomputers.

Printers

Numerous printers are available for use with microcomputers. In fact, if the appropriate interface is available, a micro can drive virtually any printer. Printers can be divided into two basic types, dot-matrix and letter-quality. Dot-matrix printers are typically faster than the letter-quality printers in a given price range; they may also include built-in features such as software-definable print fonts and pitch sizes. The dot-matrix printers receive their name from the manner in which they print characters. Each character is formed from an array of dots, rather than by a single imprint from a fully formed character (as is the case with a typical electric typewriter or letter-quality printer).

As the dot-matrix technology improves, increasing the number of dots per inch used to make characters, the distinction between dot-matrix printers and letter-quality printers will disappear. Printer technology will be covered extensively in the discussion of word processing in Chapter 5.

Monitors

There are also a number of monitors available with microcomputers. The cost of these devices ranges from $100 to $400. A monitor is slightly different from a television set; the difference lies in the ability of a monitor to provide more distinct images of finely drawn characters rather than just pictures. Monitors are also called CRTs (*cathode ray tube* refers to the picture tube itself).

Telecommunications

Another output device available to microcomputer users is the telecommunications device. The impact of these devices will be explored in other chapters; here we will examine only their function and features.

The purpose of the telecommunications device is to allow the microcomputer to communicate with other computers using telephone equipment. Micros can be used to "talk with" other microcomputers or with mainframes. They can be used to send programs or data to another machine ("upload") or to receive programs or data from another machine ("download"). They can also be used to convert the micro into a terminal that can be used with a distant machine. The resulting terminal would be called a "smart" terminal, because of its ability to download data and manipulate it locally.

SOCIAL ASPECTS OF COMPUTER TECHNOLOGY

Personal computers are very similar to mainframes in the way they are designed; they differ dramatically in the ways that they are used.

By the 1950s, the technology of the computer had become affordable and of interest to large corporations. The primary purpose of these computers was "number crunching," that is, the processing of enormous quantities of numerical data. The first software was therefore of an engineering, demographic, or military nature.

Some writers have speculated that, had the computer been developed as an adjunct to other social tasks (rather than the military or demographics), the computer would be seen in a different light. The value of the computer as a decision-making tool, as an analyst, would have been seen at an earlier stage of its development. Nevertheless, with the advent of the personal computer, people with vastly different backgrounds have become involved with computers and the result has been an explosion in the number of uses for computer power. These additional uses will key on increasing the "intelligence" of the program and its ability to aid in analysis in the social sciences that are having an increasing effect on business (e.g., industrial psychology). Also, the development of programs that respond to natural language questions about a set of data (e.g., "How many staff assistants are paid more than $15,000 per year?") will bring even more people into the computer field.

Another facet of computers worth exploring is that of the social and corporate rituals that surround the mainframe computer. The computer priesthood, with its attendant acolytes of technicians and programmers, was created by an inherently secretive industry as a result of the needs of executives everywhere to have the Absolute Truth about the last quarter's financial condition as well as an oracular statement regarding the company's production future. These unusual customs derive directly from the following salient facts about computer power in the 1950s and 1960s: (1) It was very expensive; (2) It provided a service that was unobtainable at a lower cost; and (3) It satisfied the human desire to surround and protect the important.

Most people think about computers with viewpoints that were established during this period of mainframe capacity: computers are difficult to approach (no laymen at the altar), they must be consulted through middlemen (the programmer-priests), prayers are rarely answered correctly on the first try (the computer moves in mysterious ways its wonders to perform).

The differences between mainframes and micro capabilities were discussed briefly in Chapter 1 with respect to the most efficient performance of functions. It is interesting to note that there are great differences between the two in the way that micros are regarded. For example, the micro is more approachable from a physical point of view; it is not as intimidating as a room full of components. Once neophytes have gotten over an initial uneasiness, they tend to feel more in control of the machine. If something is not going right, they can just shut it off and start over.

In addition, because the software that is available is relatively simple to use, the transition from a "Gee, that's interesting" point of view to a "Mind if I try" attitude takes place rather quickly. This software is, of course, designed to please individual business users and it presents a user environment accordingly. Most users are easily hooked into spending more time than they ordinarily might in systematizing their operation so that it might be computerized efficiently.

The Arrival of the Minicomputer

In the evolution of the computer industry, control of the mainframe resource became a vital issue in corporate politics; in most large organizations, it still is. However, a new wrinkle appeared in the late 1960s and early 1970s that started to change the perceptions of users: the so-called minicomputer.

Minicomputers performed all of the functions of a mainframe at a lower cost. Typically these were performed more slowly, and with a less elaborate array of peripheral devices. However, minicomputers also had a smaller and more approachable staff.

These machines came to serve two basic functions: that of a major computer for firms too small to afford a mainframe and that of a small special-purpose machine for a specific department within a large organization. The firms purchasing the minis for the purpose of having a major computer soon developed a corresponding (if less impressive) priesthood. However, the second function was new; it tended to take power from the control of the data processing area and made everyone else want one for their own.

These minis were, in a sense, a step backward in computer evolution in that many of them were sold as specific purpose machines; they were often purchased with a single function in mind. This specificity of purpose often takes the form of dedicated machines such as word processors.

However, these machines were more approachable and had fewer restrictions on their use. They were not in a sealed environment and were used by personnel with little formal computer training.

The Arrival of the Microcomputer

The first microcomputers were introduced in the early 1970s. For the most part, they were not products aimed at a particular market. Because of the relatively high cost of the components and the absence of the necessities of a complete computer system (i.e., operating systems software), the early micros were primarily used by hobbyists.

These first micros were developed as a result of the movement toward distributed data processing. A large computer system typically consisted of a main (controlling) processor and a number of slave devices (e.g., printers, terminals, and tape drives). Distributed data processing provides greater flexibility to perform many processing functions in locations that are physically distant from a computer.

As these peripheral devices became more sophisticated, the controlling programs for these devices became more complex. Many of these early controlling devices were hardwired, that is, the hardware was designed and built to be capable of only one function. The advantage of such a device is that it generally has the best performance (because of the specificity of the design); however, it is also the most expensive kind of device to develop.

Eventually, the idea of a controlling device that could be "programmed" came into being. The first programmable controlling device was an 8 bit microprocessor designed for a computer terminal. Because the system is often modified during product development, the development costs are less, even though the performance is not quite as good as one would expect from a hardwired device specifically designed for the purpose. These devices were a miniature version of the larger system; they were computers within a computer.

The manufacturer did not realize until at least a year later that there existed a profound potential in these small controlling devices. When the market for personal computers was discovered and defined, the chips were redesigned to allow for this function. The first microprocessor designed for a personal computing function was the Intel 8008.

TODAY'S MICROCOMPUTER

When comparing mainframe computers and micros, it is important to remember that they are based on the same principles and perform the tasks assigned to them in a similar way. The primary differences have to do with the following: speed and size (in terms of the number of variable capacity, the size of the "universe" dealt with).

Speed

The typical microcomputer is capable of executing instructions at a rate of about one million per second; some microprocessors, like the one in the Apple Macintosh, are capable of rates as high as 7.8 million per second. That is, the computer can process that many instructions in that period of time. This means all program steps, including the complex instructions required to carry out the processes of addition, subtraction, transcendental functions, and program steps.

Size

Most of the micros use an 8 bit "word" to perform their work. Some 16 bit and even 32 bit micros are coming into use. The difference between these different bit sizes can be compared to a messenger who can deliver 8 packages at a time versus one capable of carrying 16 or 32 at once. Given that they can perform the same number of trips per second, a "16 bit" messenger will carry more packages over time than an "8 bit" messenger.

The bit size of a processor is also important because, as we have seen, the amount of internal RAM memory that can be directly accessed by a computer is determined by the processor used. The trend in microcomputing is to provide software with more complex features, as well as a more user-friendly environment. The effect of these new attributes is to increase the size of the software program; the bigger the program, the larger the RAM space needed to accommodate it. For example, the typical application program for the Apple Lisa computer takes up from 200,000 to 400,000 bytes of space in the machine; this is one of the major reasons for using the Motorola 68000 processor which is capable of addressing the Megabyte (1,000K bytes) of memory in the Lisa.

The workspace of the most widely used microcomputers is 64K bytes, that is, 65,536 8 bit words that can be used for programs and data; machines with up to 512K bytes are coming into greater use. Most micros have a significant amount of this space taken up by the following functions:

1. The program language. If the micro is programmable in BASIC, for example, there must be a machine language program in the computer that will interpret the program statements in the language that the computer's processor understands. This program typically takes up about 16,000 bytes of space in a 64K machine.
2. The disk operating system. This is another program, or set of instructions, that the computer uses to interpret the commands used by the operator to store and retrieve data on mass storage devices (such as disk drives). This program typically takes up about 10,000 bytes in a 64K machine.
3. The screen memory. This is the part of the computer's workspace that is used to display data to the user of the system. The contents of this space are reproduced directly on the screen of the CRT. This space accounts for about 2,000 bytes, depending on screen size.

Additional optional functions that take up memory space are the following:

1. Graphics screens. This function allows the display of graphic information. It requires approximately one byte for each point on the graph. A 200 by 200 point graphic array takes up approximately 8,000 bytes in a 64K machine.
2. Input buffers. These are spaces set aside in the machine to temporarily store information pending transfer to some other part of the system.

Typically, a 64K microcomputer has approximately 36K bytes of space left for programs; recall that this space is for both the program and the data needed to run the program. Compare this size with the typical spaces utilized in many mainframe programs, which are often measured in hundreds of thousands of bytes. The microcomputer programmer has to learn to either limit the size of the task or to divide it up into tasks that can be handled in a smaller space.

A useful analogy is that of a man who has to perform a number of tasks but is restricted in how much he can do at a given time by the size of his desk. Suppose his desk is just big enough to hold a piece of paper for results, a sheet for scratch calculations, a sheet for instructions, and four sheets for information. To obtain additional sheets of information, or to have more results, he must pick up several sheets, walk across the room to a file cabinet, take new sheets out, and leave enough sheets in the file cabinet to make room on the desk. Obviously, the person who assigns work to this man has to keep the size of his desk in mind. The "programmer'' would have to understand that, without advance planning, the man will spend most of his time walking back and forth across the room to the file cabinet rather than sitting at his desk working.

The analogous problem in computing is that of storing and retrieving data from storage. It takes many times longer to move data from place to place if an external mass storage device is used.

Compare this situation with that of a man who has a whole conference table to spread his work out on and therefore makes fewer trips to the file cabinet, and you have an accurate analogy of the mainframe and the smaller micro. This is not to say that the two men are not capable of performing the same task, but it will clearly take the man with the small desk longer.

There are also limitations on the tasks that you might assign to the man with the smaller desk and smaller pieces of data, given the time limitations that exist in the real world. A useful comparison may be found in the actual example of a program, written to run on a micro, to perform a series of calculations on a set of meteorological data. The program took approximately 20 hours to run on the micro. The same program executed on the mainframe computer was completed in a little less than half a second. Clearly, if you were preparing a forecast for the six o'clock news on the basis of data received at 5:30, your micro would not do the job for you.

Cost

Micros can be divided according to cost into the following three groups: low-range machines ($100-$500), medium-range machines ($500-$5,000), and high-range machines ($5,000+).

Low-Range Micros

Many microcomputers in the low range have appeared. They are perhaps the most familiar because of their high visibility on television and in stores. The major limitations of these machines lies in the storage space available to them. Most rely on a tape recorder to store and retrieve data, not a very satisfactory method for mass data storage because of the low rate of data transfer. Also, the technology is not specifically designed for the needs of computer data storage. At best, these machines may be used for training in programming by writing simple programs. They may also be used to advantage as calculators that perform a series of calculations on limited data, calculations that may be too complex or repetitive for use on an ordinary calculator.

Note that many of the programmable calculators in this price range fall within the same limits of usability. The reason is that they are fundamentally identical machines. The differences lie in the full size keyboard, connections to TV sets, and availability of 80 column printers and mass storage devices that approach usability in the business environment.

The usefulness of game machines (those without a keyboard, using a joystick to interact) is extremely limited. However, this may not always be true. The primary advantage of having a keyboard lies in its usefulness in entering a range of alphanumeric information. If a program consists largely of choices to be made by the user (e.g., insert this word or that word, perform one of the listed manipulations), a joystick would provide an ideal way of choosing between alternatives on the screen. In fact, the mouse used by some of the latest micros implements just this sort of system. It is possible to perform major manipulations of existing data just by choosing different items from menus.

Typically, the low-end machines have extremely small RAM space available, 4K–16K, which may be expandable to 32K. The size of a program, and of the data that it may work with at a given time, is correspondingly limited. These machines also have a small software base, and the programs that do exist are generally very simple in nature.

Some small machines (Commodore's VIC-20, to mention one) also have a telecommunication capability at a reasonable additional cost. The small machine can then emulate a computer terminal at a considerable cost savings over most terminals. The sole limitation has to do with the short screen line length of the small machine, which is typically from 24 to 32 characters.

Medium-Range Micros

The medium-range machines, those from $500 to $5,000, represent the category most used in business. Apple, TRS 80, Commodore, and IBM Personal Computer all fall roughly into this range. The cost of the basic unit itself is generally $1,000 to $1,500; the additional cost is due to the use of peripheral devices acceptable in the business world. Some examples are letter-quality or production printers, CRTs, and mass storage devices.

These machines typically have considerably more memory, in the 64K–512K range, which is the maximum number of memory cells addressable by the microprocessors used.

There is, however, a growing number of machines on the market that feature 16 and 32 bit processors capable of handling over one million bytes (1 Megabyte). The IBM Personal Computer can theoretically handle this many, although the machine is actually limited to 512K of memory. The

Apple III, although it uses a modified 6502 processor, has an operating system capable of handling 256K bytes. Because of their larger memory capacity, they have a larger variable capacity, and their degree of usability with some programs involving the establishment of a large data base in the RAM of the computer (e.g., spreadsheet programs) is enhanced.

Apple's latest entry into the micro market, the Macintosh, has all of these capabilities. The Macintosh (Mac) is an unusual computer in several respects. It combines the great user friendly approach of the Lisa, at a much lower cost. It is also a very small machine, having a "footprint" not much larger than a sheet of notebook paper. It uses a high resolution 9 inch monitor with black characters on white background for most applications, with 128K of internal RAM, and a 400K microfloppy disk drive.

A number of applications programs are already available, including word processing, spreadsheets, and data base management. At present, due to the 128K internal space, most programs have no more space open to the user than is found in a small IBM PC, or an Apple IIe, for example. However, as soon as the chips become available, the two 64K RAM chips will be replaced with 256K chips, thus raising the space available to 512K. Also, an increase in disk drive capacity from 400K to 800K is expected.

An additional feature of the Mac that makes it very attractive is that it is highly transportable. The main unit, keyboard, and mouse weigh only 25 pounds, and a handy carrying case is available if the user wants to take it home overnight. Also, the Lisa has been redesigned to be fully compatible with all Mac software; that is, the Lisa is capable of emulating a Macintosh.

This group of computers also has the largest available software selection of the micros. The software market for these machines has thousands of individual programs for each of the older machines. The most highly developed sections of the market involve the areas of accounting, budget analysis and planning, word processing, and (of course) video games. These areas (except for video games) are discussed in detail in the following chapters.

In many cases, the software that is available will determine the hardware that is purchased. Many users continue to purchase machines at the top end of the price spectrum ($1,500 per base unit) rather than the lower-priced machines ($500) solely because of the greater software market.

The middle-range machines also have the largest range of peripheral devices available. The variety of devices and the extremely competitive market came into being as a result of an unusual marketing approach by Apple Computer. Apple decided from the outset that it would concentrate on marketing the basic unit and make information regarding the computer (and how to design peripherals for it) easily obtainable. This approach is in contrast to that of other major computer makers (indeed, most manufacturers) in that Apple gave up this share of the computer market in the hope that many people would design for their machine, thus making it more attractive.

The validity of this strategy has been borne out, both in terms of success for Apple and the fact that the same strategy was imitated by IBM when it introduced the IBM Personal Computer.

However, numerous manufacturers build many different system components. Because components can be combined to make a system, a greater degree of knowledge is required on the part of the user. The user must make certain that all of the parts of the system work together. Some of the problems to watch for are the following:

- Software package is not compatible with computer. Several of the major computers use different microprocessors, each with its own instruction set; they require individually tailored programs.
- Software requires a special peripheral device or card. Many word processing systems for the Apple, for example, require that the user purchase a special board that gives the Apple the capability to display 80 columns.
- Software is not compatible with peripheral. An example would be a graphics program that will give you pictures on the screen but cannot print them out because you lack a printer that will perform this function.

High-Range Micros

The high-range machines include a number of systems specifically aimed at the business user. North Star and Cromemco are two of the better-known companies; their systems are characterized both by the resemblance to mainframe concepts and the fact that they produce their own series of peripheral devices.

The software base for this group is relatively small, if you consider only programs written for these machines specifically. The Apple III, for example, deals with this problem by providing an emulation mode that allows the use of programs written for the Apple II.

It should be noted that the medium-range machines also support programs written for mainframe computers, particularly through the CP/M operating system. This operating system was in use long before the advent of microcomputers, and there is a huge library of available software.

The medium-range machines enter the higher-cost bracket when the user requires certain special capabilities. For example, if you want to have both letter-quality printing and the capacity to produce a large number of words per minute, you may have to spend more on the printer than you did on the rest of the computer system.

Similarly, if you wish to store millions of bytes of information in an easily accessible way, a hard disk drive will be of great value. However, the cost of the hard disk may also be greater than the initial cost of your entire microcomputer system.

There are, however, several new arrivals in the high-end bracket of personal computing that are of particular interest to the manager; they were introduced by the two companies likely to dominate the personal computer market in the 1980s—Apple Computer and IBM.

IBM's entry into this part of the computer market has been made with the IBM XT personal computer. This computer is actually an enhanced and fully loaded version of the IBM Personal Computer (PC), using the same 16 bit 8088 processor. It has a standard memory of 128K, expandable to 512K; mass memory storage is provided by a 360K floppy disk drive and a 10Mbyte hard disk. The cost of a fully loaded XT, including graphics, is approximately $7,500.

The XT also has a large software base, including programs developed for the PC. All of the standard software offerings are available in several versions, including word processors and data base managers. Another very attractive feature for business users is that the XT is compatible with the IBM mainframes now in use; IBM dominates the mainframe computer market.

The Apple entry into the high-end business market is the Lisa computer. Although it competes in the same market as the XT, it is a radically different kind of machine, offering a different environment for the computer user. It uses a 32 bit MC68000 processor, with a standard 1,000K internal memory. Mass memory is provided by a 3½ inch, 400K microfloppy disk drive and a 5 Mbyte hard disk. The cost of the standard hardware is approximately $7,000.

The most remarkable feature of the Lisa is the extraordinary environment that is presented to the user. Rather than using the usual conventions for working with a computer (that is, asking for a certain program on a certain device), the Lisa uses icons, or pictures, to represent files, devices, and programs. If you want to use the word processing program, you use the mouse to point to the LisaWrite icon, and the computer finds the program and places it on the screen, which can be thought of as a computerized desktop. Compare this with the more usual microcomputer method of typing something like "RUN WP Program, S5, D1"; in this case, a detailed knowledge of the inner structure of the machine is needed (i.e., that the word processing program is located in disk drive 1, with its controller card in slot 5). If you didn't understand that last statement, you are probably one of the great number of people who have been less than thrilled with the prospect of having to learn a lot about computers when all you want to do is use them.

With the Lisa it is also possible to place a number of different functions on the screen at the same time. For instance, you could run word processing, graphics, and spreadsheet programs simultaneously, with each application taking up its own little corner, or "window," on the screen.

The Lisa environment is also very highly integrated; that is, calculations from the LisaCalc spreadsheet program can be directly transferred to the LisaGraph program for graphing.

It is interesting to note that a similar package of programs is available for the IBM XT; however, it does not have the sort of comfortable environment presented by icons instead of filenames.

Although the Lisa and the IBM XT compete in the same market, they accomplish their computing tasks in a very different way. The Lisa is really a thinly disguised minicomputer, with a far greater potential power than any other microcomputer.

The Microcomputer Market

These computers are also interesting to look at if you want to discern the direction that computers are heading. It seems certain that computer users will want computers that are easy to use (without having to learn a lot about the machines themselves) and that provide a high degree of integration among different functions. In order to do this, the software for these machines will have to be larger; the average software program written for the Apple II and the IBM PC is about 30,000 bytes; the average-sized Lisa program is approximately 300,000 bytes. The programs of the future will certainly require computers with a large internal memory to run them. This fact will, in turn, eventually make obsolete computers with processors that can address only small internal memory spaces.

Prospective business users, particularly those who are used to the services provided by mainframe computers, should be aware that the micro business is relatively new; it has problems that are typical of a young market. In the newer companies, there may be problems with product support and documentation and with the promised versus actual capability of the new hardware or software offered. The question of whether all of your system components will work with each other, i.e., whether they are compatible, has two opposing forces that are holding the size of the problem roughly constant. On the one hand, individual companies are coming to grips with the problem, partly through the contributions of individual users. On the other hand, the fact that dozens of new peripheral devices and software products appear every month tends to negate the progress made by more established firms. By and large, the situation is improving. Also, the fact that micros have gained a foothold in the office market has improved the industry as a whole. Because companies are now dealing with persons of greater computer sophistication, software and hardware have to live up to these higher expectations. The entry of large corporations into the micro market is also adding to the push for a greater degree of professionalism in hardware and software.

Just as the microcomputer industry has spawned large numbers of peripheral devices for the basic hardware, a number of specialized software packages have also come on the market. Although it is true that microcomputers are, indeed, just like the mainframe machines, they do have special characteristics that require attention from the programmer.

Programming Disadvantages

The disadvantages faced by the programmer (and potential user) of microcomputers are as follows:

1. The main memory of the machine is typically on the order of 64K to 256K bytes; the mainframe user has a much larger space available.
2. The mass storage method used is typically the floppy disk; most floppies have a maximum storage of about 200K bytes.
3. The programming language available may not be a full implementation as used on mainframes.
4. There is a lack of large libraries of functions available on mainframes.

The first disadvantage, that of limited memory, is becoming less and less true every day. As we have seen, a number of high-end micros have appeared; these machines can handle from 256K bytes to 1,000K bytes of internal memory. However, there is no question that micros offer a smaller workspace to the user. The penalty paid is one of time; the programmer must determine a way of chopping a task into pieces, which is always more time consuming.

This "problem" of size is relative; many departments or units within the hospital will fit easily into the microcomputer environment. We must recall that the "big" mainframes that revolutionized business in the 1960s contained very little internal memory. The original IBM 360 model 40 (circa 1966) had only 64K to 128K of internal (or core) memory. Also, this size space is ideal for many applications by individual users.

The only way to effectively deal with the problem is to provide a mass storage unit that is capable of fast data transfer and storage. The hard disk drives are traditionally used for this purpose; with the lower prices of these devices resulting from the development of the smaller hard disks, they will be available to more business users. Another option is that of the solid state storage devices; if a bubble memory or RAM space of 100K–200K bytes of this fast storage is set aside, piecemeal problem solving is easily done. If a suitable way of transferring the pieces of a job is found, this disadvantage is no longer noticeable.

Mainframe programmers often complain about the lack of "civilized" languages available on micros; a reasonable response to this criticism is that many mainframe languages are indeed available on microcomputers. The following is a partial list of the languages available on today's micros:

BASIC	COBOL
FORTRAN	LOGO
Pascal	FORTH
ALGOL	

If these languages are not enough, one can always console the hardcore mainframe programmer by pointing out that with the addition of a modem (telecommunications device) all of the mainframe capabilities desired are just a phone call away. As for the absence of a large library of special routines, these special programs, dealing with statistics, graphics, and specialized formatting of data, are currently being recreated and improved for use on microcomputers.

Programming Advantages

There are definite advantages to programming a micro. The main one is that the microcomputer provides a small, manageable environment for both the programmer and the user. This "personal" aspect is one of the outstanding features of the machines. Micros are "stand-alone" systems; they are not dependent on special work environments, large staffs, or stifling conventions regarding their use.

The personal aspect of these machines extends to the cost of running programs on them as well. Spreadsheet programs, for example, were developed specifically for microcomputers; they are unique to micros. One reason that this concept was never implemented on a mainframe is that the spreadsheet program, with its emphasis on multiple use (playing "what if" with an established model), is antithetical to the maxims governing the use of large machines. As we have seen, the high cost of mainframe computer time led to strict rules governing mainframe use. Reports were carefully prepared and every routine in the program was analyzed to be sure that no precious instants of CPU time were wasted in completing a task. And the tasks to be completed? Always the conservative annual, quarterly, monthly reports—the dinosaurs of modern business. In this static conception of the business world, there is no place for a program that might be developed, used, and discarded in an afternoon, a common enough occurrence in the real world of hospital administration today.

SOFTWARE

The business software available for microcomputers fits into the following categories:

- spreadsheet programs
- word processing programs
- data base management programs
- scheduling/project management programs
- graphics programs
- utility programs

Let us examine these categories individually and determine the range of possibilities open to the business user who has neither the time nor the inclination to program micros.

Spreadsheet Programs

The spreadsheet program provides an electronic equivalent of an ordinary balance sheet. It is composed of cells that are arranged in columns and rows. Each cell can hold a label, a number, or a formula that refers to other cells containing numbers. Spreadsheet programs, which will be examined in detail in Chapter 4, are perhaps the easiest to learn, and offer the quickest return on a brief time investment, of any of the programs to be considered.

Simply put, any balance sheet that you now have can be made "intelligent" in the sense that it can do its own arithmetic operations without your help. A simple spreadsheet can become a model simulating the situation encapsulated in the sheet. By simply changing the numbers in selected areas to simulate any change in cost or activity, and pressing a button, you will cause all the formulas to be reevaluated and a new bottom line will be produced.

There are a number of special functions available for spreadsheet programs, including average, minimum or maximum, and sum of a range of numbers. All arithmetic functions are of course provided; they give the capability for extensive formulas for each cell.

Word Processing Programs

The concept of word processing is simply that it is more economical to type text into a machine display and check for errors before printing it out. This saves correction time, retyping time, not to mention paper and user frustration.

Some of the word processing programs available are direct descendants of the dedicated word processors that have been on the market for years; others have been designed especially for micros. These programs will be discussed in detail in Chapter 5.

Data Base Management Programs

Data base management programs perform the general functions of data base management, that is, they allow the user to define a record to be kept and then do all of the work necessary to store the information on a disk, recall it, and change it with just a few keystrokes.

Strictly speaking, all of the programs mentioned thus far perform a DBM task; spreadsheet and word processing programs store files that have been created during the use of the program. However, the express purpose of a DBM program is to manipulate the information in certain ways, to sort by some characteristic, for example, or to prepare reports based on very large bases of numbers or text. The program accomplishes this task by allowing the user to define fields of data that can be stored and later manipulated independently or in concert with the other pieces of information.

For example, the following information might be gathered about patient stay:

1. Registration number
2. Time of admission
3. Date of admission
4. Time of discharge
5. Date of discharge

This information could be used to determine length of stay and patient days. It could also be used to determine a pattern of admission and discharge times for a particular patient unit. Most of the DBM packages available are capable of storing at least 1,000 records as defined above; there are programs available that can store up to 65,000 records on a microcomputer.

Scheduling Programs

Another example of a generalized program to perform tasks assigned by the user is the scheduling program. There are two types: the first performs a calendar function (that is, it keeps track of appointments or tasks in a typical format); the second provides a schedule of projects or tasks, based on information about each project task. A typical program would ask you to define the overall project and then the kinds of labor that will be used to complete it. Each task is then defined in terms of the following: time required for each task, dependence on other tasks, and labor of each type required. This program will then provide a PERT chart of the entire job, as well as summaries of the jobs involved and other data entered. There are programs available that will provide Gantt charts as well.

All of the programs that have been examined thus far are general in nature; their use, the programming of the final form, is determined completely by the user. If the user does not have a clearly defined purpose in mind, the program does not offer any guidance on how to proceed on a particular problem. Thus, they are not the sort of program that will prompt for appropriate information; they are not very user friendly in that sense. They are, however, a great boon to the creative person who does not have the time or inclination to do his or her own programming in order to make use of micros. They are generalized problem-solving tools.

Graphics Programs

Graphics programs are also available to the microcomputer user. These programs take advantage of the fine graphics capabilities of microcomputers by allowing the user to input ordered strings of data and then graph the result.

The graphics programs can plot with hundreds of points in a number of different formats: line graphs, bar graphs, pie charts, scatter diagrams, hi-lo charts. Also, they typically have extensive labeling capabilities to allow the user to provide professional quality graphic analysis.

Some of these programs also have additional capabilities to allow the user to manipulate the data bases prior to graphing them. For example, given the appropriate expense versus budget figures, an additional set of data points could be prepared by asking for a cumulative or running total of expense and budget for each month.

As we have seen, one of the major trends in software development will be in the area of integrating existing functions (e.g., spreadsheets and word processing) so that they "talk to each other" more conveniently. Historically, each function evolved independently; however, the ability to easily move a graph to a word processed memo, for example, is now available to business users.

Utility Programs

As we have seen, telecommunications software allows the user to make a micro perform like a terminal and access remote computers. Other utilities available include software to update and file diskettes and copy files from one disk to another.

THE IMMEDIATE FUTURE

One of the most difficult decisions that managers and administrators will have to make with respect to computer purchases relates to the future uses of the machine. Throughout this book, we have taken care to present applications that can make full use of the computer systems that are presently in use and will continue to be of use in the foreseeable future. The technologies presently under development will not produce any new kinds of peripherals; they will only produce the same devices in use at the present time, but they will be smaller, cheaper, and faster.

The greatest advance will be seen in the area of software available to the business user. The present software will be made friendlier and will have more functions available. In this respect, the future of software will parallel the development of the hardware to run it. However, future buyers will pay more attention to the environment presented by a system rather than outstanding individual characteristics. That is, instead of being sold on a system because it has a single great program that runs on it (for example, many Apple IIs were sold because of the VisiCalc spreadsheet program), the buyer will be attracted to a system of integrated software that includes all of the options presently offered in individual programs. As we have seen, several products are already available that begin to address this need.

One aspect of personal computers that we have not yet explored is the portability of these systems. All of the microcomputers on the market today are obviously more portable than their predecessors, which required a specially trained staff to move them even from one room to another.

However, although modern systems are more easily moved than those with similar capabilities from the past, there is a difference between the ability to move a system yourself and true portability. A portable system should have the following characteristics:

- significant internal memory (at least 64K)
- readable display with at least 24 by 40 character screen output
- a built-in mass storage system (at least 128K)
- rechargeable battery power
- a built-in telecommunication system
- low weight (no more than five to ten pounds)

At the present time, the only system that fits these criteria costs approximately $10,000. However, this system's high cost is primarily due to the use of a large plasma flat screen display used as a monitor and 256K of bubble memory, both state of the art features that are still very expensive.

There are, however, several systems that are available at a much lower cost ($1,000–$2,000 range) that fit most of the above qualifications. They typically use limited displays of the Liquid Crystal Diode (LCD) type, with only four or eight lines of 32 to 40 characters each. Such displays are an excellent way of making a system truly portable and battery powered; they are very lightweight and use very little power.

The only barrier to an effective, and low-cost, portable system is that of mass storage. At present, tape recorders using microcassettes are the only low-cost system. This will probably remain the best low-cost system for the near future. However, as costs decline for such solid state devices as bubble memory and low power consumption ICs based on CMOS technology, portable systems that use them will come into widespread use.

It is difficult to predict the details of the profound effect this kind of system will have on the way business is done. Consider the following scenario, which is possible today. A supervisor, manager, or administrator has a large quantity of data immediately available at meetings, in the office, or at home. The information includes an up-to-date calendar of appointments and meetings and a complete data base on operational activity and revenue/expense. The storage system also contains the text of memos, reports, and observations by staff relevant to the meetings or business of that day.

Because the telecommunications device provides instant access to a larger data base, hospital computer systems will have to be more accessible to a larger number of staff members. The services offered by a centralized system could include complete data on operations and activity, including data as recent as the last entry made anywhere in the data net within the hospital.

Administrative decisions on issues as diverse as bed allocation and whether or not a supervisor can let a clerk go home early without disrupting the work flow can be made wherever the administrator or supervisor may be, on the basis of data received over the phone. Systems simulation programs would take the available data, project the likely outcome of a decision, and advise the user on the best manner in which to proceed. These are only a few examples of the myriad decisions that will be handled more efficiently and effectively in the future, thanks to the advent of low-cost computing power offered by microcomputers.

Chapter 3

Microcomputers in the Health Care Environment

In the last chapter, the basic components of microcomputers were introduced, along with the manner in which they interact with each other. In this chapter, we will explore the uses for microcomputer systems in the hospital management environment. Although the specific system requirements for selected uses of computer power will be explored in depth by application in succeeding chapters, it is essential first to discuss the problem in a more general way.

IS THE MICROCOMPUTER FOR YOU?

In making a decision about whether or not to expend limited financial and personnel resources on microcomputing, there are a number of issues to be considered. The options available, in the form of many combinations of hardware and software, seem endless; and as if the present profusion of systems were not confusing enough, the literature is full of reports on companies promising to make the system you have just purchased obsolete within the next six months.

For the user who is familiar with mainframe systems or dedicated minicomputers, there are several key distinctions to be made with respect to microcomputers.

First, there are relatively few turnkey microcomputer systems; for example, there is no financial analysis "system" that can be purchased. Instead, the user would have to piece together the hardware and software needed. Most of the software available for the micro market consists of individual tools, such as word processing capability, graphic capability, etc. It is up to the user to define the problem, select the appropriate "tools," gather and enter the data, and produce the report. From a formalistic point of view, the local user performs all of the functions of a data processing department at his or her own level, from system definition to supervising final report production.

This is quite different from the environment provided by a good DP department; indeed, some DP managers feel uneasy about department level computing more for these ancillary matters (i.e., system development and maintenance) than for any other reason. However, a large-scale formal effort is not required for many of the relatively small tasks for which micros are ideal. Later in this chapter we will explore some of these DP functions that must be picked up by the user.

Second, microcomputers are not (generally speaking) designed to be used by more than one person at a time. They are personal work stations that are extremely useful on a purely stand-alone basis. It is not necessary to link a micro to a larger machine or data base to perform such tasks as financial and activity analysis, word processing, and other functions. However, if the user requires a large data base that is shared between a number of departments, communication with a centralized computer system is certainly most desirable.

The most important objective to keep in mind while considering the purchase of a microcomputer system is a simple one: its intended use. The many options available pose a real problem; there is no "standard" system for use in business. The best approach is to get some idea of what a simple system can do and then vary the peripheral devices one at a time to get an idea of the larger possibilities. It is also important to consider the impact that a microcomputer will have on your staff, both in terms of new capabilities provided and the price that must be paid in development time and training.

SELECTING THE MICROCOMPUTER

Although there is no clearly defined standard system, the following shopping list is a good start:

Hardware

- 1 64–128K microcomputer with 80 column capability
- 2 disk drives
- 1 dot-matrix printer with interface card
- 1 12 inch monitor

Software

- 1 word processing program
- 1 spreadsheet program
- 1 data base manager program

If the buyer follows the guidelines for purchasing hardware and software outlined in Chapter 2, the result will be an inexpensive ($3,000), usable system. In fact, this system is typical of the starter systems purchased by many departments as their first microcomputer system. All of the applications in this book can be done on this size system, with the exception of those requiring additional software (e.g., graphics).

The only disadvantage lies in the relatively small internal memory space supplied (64–128K). As we have noted, the next few years will see a number of software applications that will require a large internal memory. However, the buyer must keep from being hypnotized by possibilities and pay attention to what can be done here and now. For example, if small spreadsheets were the major intended use, a larger system may never be needed.

The software recommended provides the three general functions preferred by most users. The word processing function alone may recoup the cost of the computer; Chapter 5 illustrates the many uses for such a system. If all you wanted was a good quality, low cost, word processing system, a 64K machine could form the base for a perfectly acceptable setup. There would be no need to spend the additional dollars on a more powerful system that was capable of addressing a larger internal memory.

Also, such a system could be enhanced with the addition of a fast letter quality printer; however, the cost of top of the line printers may be as much as the cost of the base system (approximately $2,000).

Spreadsheet programs are perhaps the most impressive general function programs available. Their power lies in the flexibility provided to the user. The electronic balance sheet or spreadsheet will tirelessly perform extensive calculations on limited volumes of data.

Adding a larger memory space to a function like this may make it more suitable for certain applications. The larger the RAM space available, the larger a spreadsheet can be. A 64K micro can handle only about 3 pages of data and analysis; a 256K machine could handle up to 15 pages.

Data base management (DBM) programs provide flexibility in storing data with the ability to manipulate the information in specific ways; sorting, some calculation, and sophisticated report generation are some of the most important features. As mentioned, larger hard disk systems can provide for all but the most extensive DBM applications.

A good analogy to keep in mind when considering acquiring a personal computer system is that of a "helper" or group of helpers to perform tedious work quickly and efficiently. There are numerous cases of reports formerly requiring days of effort by highly paid management personnel that are now being done on microcomputers by assistants or secretaries; and the reports are completed in hours instead of days.

Unfortunately, these eminently capable electronic helpers are very stupid, in that they must be given precise instructions to perform their assigned tasks. They also have limitations in terms of the amount of data that can be manipulated.

What Do You Want To Do?

As we have seen, the limitation of microcomputer programs can be defined in terms of the following: (1) the internal memory (RAM) available, (2) the external memory (mass storage, e.g., disk drives) available, and (3) the actual algorithms in the program itself. When considering a microcomputer program, the buyer should determine whether or not the program is RAM based, that is, whether the program is dependent on the size of the internal memory for what it will do. Many word processing programs allow you to work with a piece of text no bigger than the internal space of the machine itself.

In the case of a word processing program, this limitation may not be a problem. However, if you want to run a data base management program with many hundreds of large records, it is essential that the program be disk based; that is, the internal memory of the machine is used only as a space for program instructions and as a workspace for a particular record being accessed at a given time. When dealing with a disk-based system, it will take longer to run the program than if all of the information could be loaded directly into RAM. One way to avoid the time problem is to make use of hard disks rather than floppy disks. Because the access and transfer times are so much better, the time needed to run the program may be reduced by a factor of ten or more.

As far as the actual amount of data is concerned, as we saw in Chapter 2, microcomputers can support very large external memory devices; multiple hard disk systems with up to 20 Megabytes each could be used if desired. As the 256K RAM spaces become more commonplace, storage space will cease to be a problem for all but the largest data base management tasks. It all depends on what the potential user is able to spend.

What Can the Staff Do?

When choosing a computer system, it is important to gauge the level of expertise and interest on the part of the proposed users. If, for example, your staff has several people who are creatively minded and are willing to spend some extra time, a starter system as described could be a good inexpensive choice. If, on the other hand, your staff has little or no interest in computers, the generic problem-solving software may not be the answer.

In this case, it may be necessary to take the more traditional route; i.e., ask the DP department or a consultant to take on the task of program management and system development.

Another important issue to consider is that of the existing computer capability of other hospital staff, both in terms of mainframe support and other microcomputers.

In some cases, a large DP department may exercise a great deal of control over the microcomputer to be purchased. It is essential for the local user to understand the concern felt by DP managers when individuals or departments express the desire to obtain microcomputers. This concern is often due to the belief that, sooner or later, the user will want to access the mainframe. Microcomputers, as we have seen, offer little in the way of standardized formats for data transfer, either by diskette, telecommunications, or coaxial cable. Many DP managers foresee a tremendous burden on their service from diversity at the local level.

If the user needs to have access to the mainframe and its data, it is clear that there must be a meeting of minds between the local user and the DP manager prior to the purchase of any equipment. If, however, the user needs a stand-alone system, using data gathered at a local level or from the bottom lines of standardized reports, access to the mainframe becomes a null issue and should not affect the choice of a system.

It is also helpful to take note of other microcomputer applications (if any) in your institution, both in terms of learning from mistakes and taking advantage of any developed systems or problem-solving techniques. If you know of a successful computer application that you would like to use in your area, be sure equivalent software is available on the machine you have in mind. Also, be aware that just because VisiCalc, for example, runs on both the Radio Shack TRS80 and the Apple IIe, it does not mean you can exchange disks between the two machines. Because of different disk formats, this would not be possible.

INTRODUCING THE SYSTEM

Thus far, our discussion has focused on the use of microcomputers in the general business environment. Indeed, many aspects of microcomputer use in general business are applicable in the health care setting. There are certain differences, however, that should be considered.

First, because of the highly technical nature of many of the patient care and (perhaps research) activities that are carried out in most hospitals, there is great potential that by the time hospital management decides to consider their use in a management setting microcomputers will already be present in the offices and laboratories of physicians or other members of the health care team. These micros are usually used for computing algorithms related to the calculation of test values or the manipulation of research information. Very likely, the hospital's intensive care units are equipped with sophisticated physiological monitoring equipment that is connected to microprocessors for equipment control and monitoring and to microcomputers for storage, manipulation, and analysis of patient-specific information regarding hemodynamics, pulmonary status, and cardiac status.

This environment should be useful for introducing staff members to the management uses of micros because the familiarity may reduce the anxiety often associated with the introduction of new technology. Such familiarity does not exist in the typical business setting.

The management staff might also be encouraged quite directly to use available microcomputer support. This encouragement should take the form of recognition that time has been saved and the quality of information has been improved, as well as general appreciation of a job well done (or at least done better than might otherwise have been the case). In Chapter 1, we indicated that the mere presence of a microcomputer encourages its beneficial use. We also described the steps that should be taken to make this introduction. Most managers are bright and energetic people who are usually looking for creative problem-solving tools. Introducing the microcomputer into the management environment not only provides managers with many exciting opportunities to be innovative but also sends a clear message about the institution's appreciation of the creative person. Moreover, it sends a message indicating the institution's expectations of its managers.

Of course, in introducing the micro to the hospital management setting, care should be taken to stress the importance of considering the micro as a means to an end, not as an end in itself. What matters is the production of specific management results. Many small businesses have failed because their proprietors fell under the hypnotic spell of the microcomputer and forgot to look after their business. A little "computeritis" is to be expected as novices explore the many exciting things the micro can do for them, but the slightest hint that the manager has become too fascinated with the technology of the micro should be dealt with swiftly and clearly; managers must understand that micros are just another tool in their box.

Initial Projects

Having familiarized your staff with the microcomputer, either through a formal program or by making it available with software, the next step is to provide some guidance regarding the capabilities and limits of the machine.

As we have seen, one of the distinguishing traits of the mainframe computer environment is that of an extreme degree of control over the computer. This degree of control was made necessary by the high cost of the resource and the high level of expertise needed to obtain the maximum benefit. Microcomputers, however, because of their relatively low cost and low level of expertise required, do not warrant the same degree of control.

It is helpful, particularly in terms of ensuring that people will use the machine constructively, to make assignments from the start that will allow staff members to interact with the computer in a useful and successful way. The manager or administrator can ensure that this happens by considering short-term projects that will have a quick, positive return on a small investment of time.

Spreadsheets

One such example is the spreadsheet program. This genre provides the equivalent of an electronic spreadsheet on the screen. The major system commands and functions can be learned in an afternoon. This type of program, which will be discussed extensively in Chapter 4, can be used to prepare the following kinds of reports in a short time:

- budget and activity presentations taking the form of a standardized table (e.g., calculating dollar and percent variance, cost per patient day or admission) that must be done every month. Once the blank spreadsheet has been prepared, it can be loaded and used over and over again.
- summary presentations requiring frequent revision as the final pieces of data become available. The fact that most of the information is entered into the machine makes the printing of preliminary versions easier; the math functions provided ensure accuracy.
- limited data base management relating to specific areas. For example, a supervisor may notice an expense increase in a particular expense category and may wish to compare costs and usage on an item-by-item basis over a period of months or years.

Word Processing

Another application providing immediately useful results is that of the word processing program. Discussed in detail in Chapter 5, word processing can be learned quickly (typically in an afternoon) and can provide the following useful functions:

- ongoing lists of problems or projects. Although word processing programs will not sort lists, they provide a medium for list keeping that is much easier to work with than just a pad of paper, especially if the lists have to be kept on a formal (i.e., typed) basis.
- performance plans or lists of job objectives and accomplishments. This kind of ongoing file can provide an up-to-date list of these items.
- report writing. Many managers prefer to see what they are writing while they compose a report rather than getting involved with the whole dictating, waiting for transcription, revising procedure. Typing on a word processing program provides flexibility in editing and produces immediate, typed, hard copy.
- memoranda and reports.

Once staff members are sold on the micro, guidance from higher levels may no longer be required. However, it is a good idea to ensure the productive use of the machine by assigning certain tasks to staff for placement on the micro. The application chapters that follow provide a springboard for the use of computers by a number of departments. Throughout all efforts, administrators and managers are encouraged to give staff the maximum leeway to use their own approaches in problem solving. Given the low cost of the system, the expense involved can be recouped in a single creative use.

Decentralized Data Processing

The applications considered thus far are purely "local" uses of microcomputers; that is, the program, all data, report generation, and expertise are provided at the micro itself by the user. As we have mentioned, applications that will come into increasing use are those that involve distributed data processing. These applications may be identical to those described above, except that the data base involved may be kept by the hospital mainframe and then downloaded onto the micro for manipulation.

This kind of use can provide benefits to both the local user as well as to the mainframe staff in that prospective uses of data are tested at a local level. If a particular application is found to be useful, the complete report format and algorithms can be given to the mainframe programmers, cutting down on development time. This approach would be helpful when dealing with applications that require extensive manipulation of a large data base and that provide information in a standard format with a long useful life.

However, most applications have a useful life of only about six months before some change in expectations at the department level, or in the accounting or organizational environment, make a revision necessary. Given the long length of time required to make changes in mainframe programs because of the many conventions and system requirements, many mainframe programs provide only a fraction of what is desired; a locally produced program can provide the needed reports without taxing the central resource.

This sort of local use also tends to ease the burden placed on the resource by centralized data processing departments. Given the ease of working with data at a local level, centralized data systems may come to perform a library or record-keeping function, along with that of providing selected official reports relating to patient activity and finance. All manipulation of this data would be carried out by departments, thus eliminating a perennial squabble between department heads competing for a limited resource.

The notion of a truly decentralized data processing system is not a new one, of course, but it is easy to see how the availability of computer power with a small capital investment is changing the traditional image of what a "computer system" should be. Suppose an administrator provides a microcomputer for the use of staff members, along with a small library of flexible canned software; no threat to the established order thus far. After several months of use, one of the staff assistants puts together a program that entails a large data base management effort, one that will require a secretary to enter all of the needed information. A secretary is hired and assigned to the staff assistant. Since this program proves successful, it is suggested that the program could be improved if a formal program was written to handle the data manipulation and report generation. A programmer is then hired on a temporary basis to perform this limited task and the entire project is assigned to a managerial staff person.

Each of the above steps sounds perfectly reasonable, but observe the result. This administrator now has his or her own miniature data processing department. Suppose all of the other department heads try to jump on the bandwagon? The amazing thing about microcomputers is that they are so inexpensive that the main barrier to setting up one's own DP department no longer exists. There is no "reasonable" point at which to draw the line. Perhaps, given the profusion of uses that will be required of computers for hospitals to stay competitive, and the inability of a central authority to provide these applications, no line can or should be drawn.

PROGRAMS IN ACTION

So far, the picture of microcomputing presented is a very positive one. The use of micros is, of course, not without pitfalls. An analogy can be found in the idea that the productivity of a manager can be improved by giving that person additional support staff. The problem is that if these new staff members are directed into useless activities, a great deal of useless work will take place. A computer provides the equivalent of assistants; if the wrong direction is taken, much useless paper can be generated by a machine capable of processing one million instructions per second!

In the 1950s and 1960s, the main barrier to setting up a data processing department was that of the capital cost of the machine. The cost of the computer and the annual cost of the staff needed to run it were roughly equal. Today, because of the low cost of computers, a $3,000 system may be the center of an $80,000 data base management effort comprising a secretary (data entry), several assistants (data gathering), several programmers (data formatting), and management time to coordinate the effort. That is, the cost of the hardware is insignificant compared with the personnel costs involved.

Another problem to watch for is the occasional staff member who becomes fascinated with the computer for its own sake and loses sight of the useful objective that may have been assigned. Virtually everyone passes through this phase; it is hard to keep from being impressed with what a computer can do. The problem can be handled by being more results oriented and less potential oriented; that is, give positive strokes for actual accomplishments rather than for statements such as "I could provide the following 50 permutations of such-and-such data."

Potentially serious problems can also arise with respect to the maintenance of data bases at several different levels or areas of the same organization. Two or more data bases containing the same information may start out being identical, but as time goes on they may tend to diverge until the information stored in one is no longer in agreement with the others. Reports from different areas may therefore be derived from sets of data that are dissimilar, and confusion may arise.

Traditionally, this problem has been solved by having only one data base. In a distributed data processing scheme such as the one described above, the problem may be solved by designating one area as the "official" source charged with the responsibility of making the data base available on diskettes, or over the phone.

Although there is a certain amount of time inevitably required to make all staff members experts in the use of microcomputers, it takes only a few creative uses (or individuals) to recoup the investment. Managerial or supervisory staff are not the only ones affected; once a program is up and running, it is usually turned over to a secretary or assistant. This is particularly true of programs requiring large data bases. Again, a results-oriented approach is preferred in dealing with what could be a useless profusion of data.

An additional benefit of control (or at least monitoring) of the micro resource is that duplication of effort can be avoided at the outset. Staff members will naturally imitate approaches that are successful; administrators should be careful to give positive feedback to all potentially good uses of the resource to ensure that everyone will continue to think for themselves. One way of ensuring that good approaches will not be reinvented time and again is to encourage the sharing of techniques and reports in an informal way, possibly during monthly or quarterly meetings.

Guidelines for Use

Some maintenance functions provided by centralized computer services are not apparent to the casual user; these services may need to be provided in a limited way at the local level. The following discussion pertains primarily to the typical microcomputer system that is shared by several persons (or an office or department):

- Important programs and data should be "backed up," that is, copies should be kept in a safe place. This is particularly true of the data bases and reports that are updated over a long period of time. Most data processing services do this on a weekly basis (minimum); it is a matter of personal preference in doing it at the local level. The user should consider the fact that if the data is lost, it must all be reentered from paper records, if they exist.
- The security of the system should be considered. Typically, users keep their own disks and programs at their own work area and bring them to the machine when they use them. However, this may not be true of systems that use hard disks for storage of data from different individuals or departments. Simply locking up the relevant program disks (and possibly the machine itself) is often sufficient to deal with the problem.
- Some data may require special handling. This is true of data pertaining to patient-related statistics and financial reports. Some programs may utilize data that is restricted; the hospital attorney should be consulted on these matters, if possible. Staff members having computers at home

should be given guidance on whether or not to take this data home to work on reports.

- Scheduling of time on the system is a good practice. A signup sheet should indicate the user's name, time, and purpose for using the machine. This sheet serves the additional purpose of keeping administrators informed about the use of the resource.
- Canned software use must be supervised. Purchased (or "canned") software can be very expensive, often costing from $200 to $500; because copies cannot typically be made by the user, the originals must be circulated. There should be a system of control for these items, especially if there is more than one machine available or if staff members have computers at home.

The above functions can be performed by a single individual under the direction of the departmental "expert." They are important enough that someone with authority should receive the task as a staff assignment.

Developing Expertise

It takes time to develop programs to solve problems. Remember that a program or system involves more than just the machines. If a major data base management effort is needed, the tasks of system definition and system development, including decisions regarding hardware and software, the data to be acquired and how it is to be stored, are all taken on by the local user. For many small tasks, a formal exercise in systems development is not necessary; for larger tasks it is helpful to avail oneself of the services of the DP department or other appropriate consultants. With practical experience you will see the development of expertise on the part of managers, supervisors, and users in programming, learning the capabilities of software, and understanding the role of the system's different components and the algorithms required to manipulate data.

The administrator should realize that not all problems are solvable by "quick fix" software (particularly the spreadsheet programs) and that the amount of time a staff person spends pursuing a computerized solution of a problem is related to activities in the following areas:

1. Learning the capabilities of the system and the software purchased to run it
2. Learning the idiosyncrasies of the system and the limits to programs and systems

3. Defining the problem to be solved (typically with the administrative superior)
4. Acquiring the necessary data
5. Finalizing the report format
6. Writing the necessary program or guiding the computer through the process of producing the required report
7. Entering the data in question
8. Producing the report itself

The least amount of time is spent on item 8; computers are very fast once they have been given their task. The administrator should be most sensitive to the needs required by items 1 and 2 and give the subordinate sufficient time, and perhaps the educational tools, to deal with learning a new system. Many computer stores and community colleges offer classes to aid the neophyte in learning how to use micros creatively; the subordinate should be encouraged to utilize this sort of resource if so inclined.

Administrators can also assist with items 3 and 5 by providing clear direction, both in terms of stating the problem and in keeping the subordinate attuned to the final goal. This prevents the sidetracking common to computer users because computers offer so many easy options to explore.

The problem represented by item 4, that of acquiring the needed data, poses a special set of difficulties. In the organizational world, information is power, and it is typically guarded by those who have it. Many departments are dependent on the activities of other areas; administrators are acutely affected by this problem. The administrator can help by using his or her influence to help the subordinate obtain required data from other departments. This problem also pops up when particularly large data bases are used.

Finally, the administrator may wish to introduce a formal method for justifying the implementation of new microcomputer applications. Such a method might include:

1. A statement of the problem
2. Expected results or reports to be generated
3. Quantifiable benefits expected
4. Costs (including system design and development, programming, data entry, and hardware and software)

The administrator may wish to institute a yearly review of the use of the system to clear out deadwood and encourage the development of useful services.

INFORMATION CENTERS

The information center is a facility, usually within the central data processing or information system, that supports users by providing a storehouse of computerized information which can be accessed for purposes such as report generation, data inquiry, and data manipulation. The users of such systems have the opportunity of utilizing valuable software tools, as well as receiving technical advice and support. Therefore, information is more accessible to the users while performing their managerial or other work.

The information center allows the user to modify reports to fit changing needs; it also permits the user to satisfy information needs that may not have been considered during information system design. The result is that the user perceives the system to be more responsive to his or her needs and the providers of the information are better able to accommodate changing needs—thus helping to avoid the friction and frustration that may otherwise exist.

In developing an information center both the information system's leadership and information users must make a number of commitments. The information system must provide applications, software, educational materials, and technical expertise so that users can easily access the system. The users must also agree to the utilization and security requirements of the system. Information systems are developed and implemented by the information system's staff who provide the technical expertise while the users provide the expertise in applications and requirements definitions.

Implementation of an information center requires a health care institution to assume a user perspective, have a clearly defined purpose and goals for the center, acquire appropriate staff and facilities, and assure confidentiality of information.

Microcomputer users will no doubt find the information center a very attractive idea. The users' enhanced ability to interact with a central data base to solve management or other problems through packaged tools and available data can only bring them closer together with other microcomputer users. A closer working relationship can also be established with the central information system.

The information center can assist the department manager who is faced with a decision involving the analysis of computer resource needs. It can provide expert advice on the best mix of hardware and software to accomplish the tasks at hand.

In addition, the center can provide a means to ensure that the organization is receiving a satisfactory return on its computer resource investment.

This can be done by establishing reasonable standards regarding the types and brands of equipment that may be linked to a larger network. Such standardization might help avoid the cost of redevelopment in cases where local computer use is established before larger scale networking. However, it is wise to avoid a heavy-handed approach that overcontrols the local user. In those cases where computer resource needs are unique and applicable to single users, departments, or other units, the information center should not be in a position of control. Control in these cases should rest with the responsible administrator.

Hospitals may find that the idea of an information center may not be perceived in the same way by all users or the users' perceptions may not agree with those of the data processing department. For example, the data processing department may believe that its responsibility carries the controlling voice in all data processing decisions. The user departments may not share this view. If they believe that their legitimate needs and efforts are being thwarted by a seemingly bureaucratic process, this can pose potentially serious problems for departments eager to acquire computer resources. On the other hand, the data processing department indeed perceives this role correctly with regard both to the development of large-scale networking of computers and information whose integrity must be protected.

It is extremely important for the institution to clearly and explicitly define the role of the information center, including its responsibility and authority, and to convey this definition to the user departments.

Information centers can provide a valuable source of information that can be shared by all small computer users in the hospital. This material may come from outside sources such as periodicals, technical books and manuals, seminars, as well as information gained through personal contacts with other institutions or in the computer industry. Information about applications developed by hospital departments may also be shared through the information center in meetings, newsletters, or the development of an applications library. We are all in this together and the more tools to help us do our jobs the better.

Chapter 4

Spreadsheet Programs

If any one kind of software can be said to have sparked the explosive growth of the use of microcomputers in the business community, it would be the spreadsheet program. In this chapter, the concept of the "electronic spreadsheet" will be explored and examples of applications to health care management will be introduced. The chapter contains numerous examples of the development and use of electronic spreadsheets in the health care setting.

At present, there are a number of spreadsheet programs available for all of the computers aimed at the business user. Among the most popular programs are VisiCalc, Lotus 1-2-3, Multiplan, Supercalc, and Visicalc, Advanced Version. There are at least 50 different versions available for different computers ranging in cost from $50 to $300. The examples in the pages that follow are implementable on any of the available programs, with little or no modification.

Electronic spreadsheet programs are based on the following simple idea; suppose the computer screen were to be made to resemble a typical columnar pad or spreadsheet. The sheet would be divided into columns and rows, with the entry marked by a coordinate according to column and row to denote a cell in memory. Another way to visualize it would be to see it as an array of cells, so many rows high by so many columns wide. When the program is running, the user sees only a portion of the total spreadsheet; the screen is like a window onto the total sheet. VisiCalc, for example, has the capability of storing 254 rows by 63 columns, depending on the memory available; the screen may show only 20 rows by 8 columns.

The obvious advantages so far are, of course, those inherent in any word processing program, namely, that modifications to the text are easily accomplished. However, the inventors of VisiCalc went one step further to include the advantages of using the computer as a calculator.

The method used for introducing the capability for calculation into the text was simple; each cell within the sheet was given a pair of coordinates; a letter to denote the column and a number to denote the row. Given the fact that each cell was unique, one merely has to program in the ability for the machine to perform the arithmetic operations. For example, if you wanted to figure the cost of a group of items, given the cost/item in cell A1 and the number of items in cell B1, the total cost could be placed in cell C1 with the formula +A1*B1.

Thus, a spreadsheet entry consists of one of the following:

1. A label
2. A number
3. A mathematical operation on the entries in some other cell (or group of cells), with the answer placed in the cell containing the formula.

FUNCTIONS

Some of the specific functions available in today's spreadsheet programs are the following:

- ordinary mathematical operations of addition, subtraction, multiplication, and division
- transcendental functions, such as sine, cosine, and tangent
- logical operations of "and," "not," "or" (used in decision making within the program)
- mean, median, largest/smallest of a given series
- column width
- format for numerical data (i.e., integer, real, dollars and cents)

Alphabetic titles, numeric values, or calculations (formulas) can be entered into each of the thousands of locations, allowing the user to create tables, charts, and records. The ability to format each location or "cell" on the spreadsheet enables you to solve problems in a fraction of the time normally spent. The program stores, or "remembers," the titles, data, and formulas you have entered and allows you to replicate them in other parts of the spreadsheet. Most important, once a spreadsheet has been set up, changes in data you have entered in one part of the spreadsheet will automatically initiate recalculations throughout the entire spreadsheet in locations that are affected by the change, including the bottom line, of course. Some spreadsheet systems provide the ability to graph information as well as to present trends.

TYPES OF PROGRAMS

Spreadsheet programs do have limits, but to explore them it is necessary to understand that there are three varieties available. The original VisiCalc implementation had the spreadsheet totally contained in the computer's RAM memory. That is, the size of the spreadsheet (how many rows and columns) was limited to the space available within the machine; this limitation was approximately 36K bytes of storage in the average 64K byte microcomputer. This translates to a sheet of perhaps 16 columns and 150 rows, depending on the complexity of calculations involved. The mid-range machines, those with memory expandable to 256K bytes, have room for up to 200K byte spreadsheets. The limitations on these machines may lie in the storage device used to keep the sheet; most disk drives have less than 200K bytes storage per disk.

The second type of spreadsheet program is the disk-based system of more recent origin. This kind of program places only a certain amount of the sheet in the computer's RAM space at a given time; the size of the spreadsheet is limited only by the size of the floppy disk used (typically 140K bytes).

The third type has a RAM-based sheet similar to the original spreadsheet program but allows the user to link a number of sheets together. VisiCalc, on the other hand, does not allow distinct sheets to "talk to each other" very well.

This size limitation places a definite boundary on the usefulness of spreadsheet programs. The major areas of application for the first type of program lie in the many daily tasks requiring 1 to 4 pages of tables, data, or analysis, or a combination of sections of this size. Machines with a larger RAM space can have a correspondingly larger sheet in memory.

SPREADSHEET CAPABILITY

The greatest advantages of the spreadsheet programs are simply stated as follows:

- They are very simple to learn and easy to use; the spreadsheet concept is familiar to everyone in business.
- They require no special programming skills.

- The format of the sheet can be changed readily, much more easily than rewriting a typical computer program.

If you can design a spreadsheet, and find your way around on the keyboard of an electric typewriter, you can use an electronic spreadsheet program.

A good example of a simple spreadsheet can be seen in Exhibit 4-1. This sheet illustrates several of the basic functions of these programs. The only real formulas entered provide the totals for each expense class and for each month.

The same sheet is expanded in Exhibit 4-2, showing a full year data base for an account. Note the smaller print size in this report. It is necessary to distinguish the limitations imposed on the size of the spreadsheet by the program, the limitations imposed by your system's memory size, and the size of the sheet that your printer will print.

Exhibit 4-1 A Simple Spreadsheet

HOSPITAL OPERATIONS
QUARTERLY EXPENSE REPORT

ACCOUNT: 10701
ACCT. NAME: UNIT 3 EAST

EXPENSE CLASS	JUL	AUG	SEPT	TOTAL
PRO & ADMIN	1750	1850	1600	5200
AFSCME	3215	3412	3153	9780
OFFICE	843	843	843	2529
OTHER PAY	0	0	0	0
UNBGT PAY	0	0	0	0
POSTAGE	23	34	43	100
TEL & TEL	1352	134	231	1717
FOOD	34	32	43	109
GEN & OFFICE	1532	1932	2132	5596
PHARMACY	1524	2142	1643	5309
LINEN	1200	1432	153	2785
MED/SURG	3214	5324	2154	10692
TOTAL	14687	17135	11995	43817

Exhibit 4-2 Expanded Spreadsheet: Full Year Data

HOSPITAL OPERATIONS
ANNUAL EXPENSE REPORT

RUN DATE:
REVISED:

ACCOUNT:
ACCT. NAME:

EXPENSE CLASS	JUL	AUG	SEPT	OCT	NOV	DEC	JAN	FEB	MAR	APR	MAY	JUN	TOTAL
PRO & ADMIN	1750	1850	1600	1850	1850	1850	1740	1200	2100	2134	1987	1765	21676
AFSCME	3215	3412	3153	2988	2786	3100	2651	1766	4214	2343	431	4599	34658
OFFICE	843	843	843	843	932	932	932	932	932	932	932	932	10828
OTHER PAY	0	0	0	0	314	215	22	0	0	0	0	0	551
UNBGT PAY	0	0	435	0	0	0	214	66	0	0	0	0	715
POSTAGE	23	34	43	32	42	52	13	24	16	54	32	12	377
TEL & TEL	1352	134	231	231	432	133	12	144	154	253	166	186	3428
FOOD	34	32	43	12	32	14	32	15	45	34	27	3	323
GEN & OFFICE	1532	1932	2132	2415	233	1456	3415	2143	633	712	3415	612	20630
PHARMACY	1524	2142	1643	2134	2166	321	3215	2134	1276	2109	312	2362	21338
LINEN	1200	1432	153	1319	2153	234	543	1425	2356	2765	1324	1789	16693
MED/SURG	3214	5324	2154	3142	514	3765	3142	2176	3812	1342	2176	412	31173
TOTAL	14687	17135	12430	14966	11454	12072	15931	12025	15538	12678	10802	12672	162390

For example, an 8½ by 11 sheet of paper, with half-inch margins, would have 7.5 inches available for printed output. If the print font used is 10 pitch (10 characters per inch), there would be room for $7.5 \times 10 = 75$ characters per line.

In the case of the spreadsheet shown in Exhibit 4-2, there are 14 columns of data. Such a report could fit on the paper with the font size described only if the columns were 5 characters wide. Obviously, the smaller characters must be used to obtain the necessary number of characters per column. Another solution to this problem can be found in purchasing a wide-bed printer, or simply turning the paper sideways.

The spreadsheet can also be divided into large areas that can be printed out as separate sheets later. Each sheet in a report may therefore use information contained on the others, given the fact that they are all present in memory. Some parts of the larger VisiCalc sheet may never be printed; these areas may be set aside for constants, scratch calculations, etc. The user is typically interested in final results.

An example of the capability of building on existing spreadsheets is shown in Exhibit 4-3, which illustrates a report based on the report in Exhibit 4-2. This report allows a manager or department head to use an inflation figure for each individual line item in a yearly account summary in order to predict expenses for an upcoming year.

The format of the sheet is identical to that of Exhibit 4-2 except that the inflation factor is entered prior to the monthly data. Keep in mind the fact that all of the numbers in Exhibit 4-3 are the result of a calculation based on the inflation factor and the data contained in Exhibit 4-2.

Once this sheet is set up, it can be easily used to provide assistance in cost projection based on available information about the rate of cost increase in individual areas. The report can be updated with new information in seconds and printed in less than a minute.

CREATING A TEMPLATE

Another use of the spreadsheet programs can be illustrated by zeroing out all of the entries on the sheet; this can be done by replacing all of the entries in Exhibit 4-2 with zeroes; the change will be mirrored throughout the sheet. This sheet is then saved to disk under a separate filename. You may wish to protect the template from change by either locking the file or placing a "write protect" tab on the disk itself. "Write protect" is computer jargon for physically prohibiting data from being "written" or stored, for example, on a disk or tape.

Exhibit 4-3 Expanded Spreadsheet: Inflation Factor

HOSPITAL OPERATIONS
EXPENSE PROJECTION
BASED ON ACTUAL FISCAL 1983

RUN DATE:
REVISED:

EXPENSE CLASS	INDEX	JUL	AUG	SEPT	OCT	NOV	DEC	JAN	FEB	MAR	APR	MAY	JUN	TOTAL
PRO & ADMIN	1.105	1934	2044	1768	2044	2044	2044	1923	1326	2321	2358	2196	1950	23952
AFSCME	1.115	3585	3804	3516	3332	3106	3457	2956	1969	4699	2612	481	5128	38644
OFFICE	1.125	948	948	948	948	1049	1049	1049	1049	1049	1049	1049	1049	12182
OTHER PAY	1.105	0	0	0	0	347	238	24	0	0	0	0	0	609
UNBGT PAY	1.105	0	0	481	0	0	0	236	73	0	0	0	0	790
POSTAGE	1.245	29	42	54	40	52	65	16	30	20	67	40	15	469
TEL & TEL	1.095	1480	147	253	253	473	146	13	158	169	277	182	204	3754
FOOD	1.035	35	33	45	12	33	14	33	16	47	35	28	3	334
GEN & OFFICE	1.115	1708	2154	2377	2693	260	1623	3808	2389	706	794	3808	682	23002
PHARMACY	1.175	1791	2517	1931	2507	2545	377	3778	2507	1499	2478	367	2775	25072
LINEN	1.115	1338	1597	171	1471	2401	261	605	1589	2627	3083	1476	1995	18613
MED/SURG	1.215	3905	6469	2617	3818	625	4574	3818	2644	4632	1631	2644	501	37875
TOTAL		16753	19756	14159	17118	12935	13848	18259	13749	17766	14384	12269	14301	185296

Once this is done, the spreadsheet program becomes a template that can now be used for any account by simply plugging in the appropriate information. Often, a first draft of a complex report may take as long to prepare with spreadsheet programs as it does by hand; the major saving in time results from these "spinoff" uses of the same sheet or data base. The fact that a spreadsheet can be edited and retyped in minutes is also a great timesaver, particularly when the sheet goes through a number of revisions before formal submission.

SUMMARY SHEETS

Spreadsheet programs are also of use to the manager or administrator who wishes to have summary sheets for accounts. Even in institutions that make summary sheets available to managers, the summaries are not always in a useful format. Exhibit 4-4 shows a typical summary sheet detailing monthly and year-to-date expense, comparison to budget, and percent variance. This sheet is based on a data base containing monthly expense and budget figures for the fiscal year considered.

This basic report can be augmented by the addition of a patient-day related budget, that is, a budget showing the amount budgeted based on the expected expense per item per patient day (see Exhibit 4-5).

The advantage of a budget comparison by patient days is that expenses related to patient days can be highlighted. This information is useful when preparing budget projections and forecasts.

This report illustrates another major use of the spreadsheet program, as an easily usable adjunct to existing mainframe reports. Typically, large data processing departments are unable to respond quickly to the transient needs of small departments within an institution.

The examples shown illustrate the usefulness of the spreadsheet programs for small-scale data base management efforts. They highlight the greatest strength of these programs, which is the ability to perform endless calculations on a relatively small group of items; in this case, between 150 and 500 pieces of data.

FINANCIAL REPORTS

Most institutions require some form of financial report on a monthly basis; the time available to produce these reports is necessarily limited. However, once the report format is entered into the computer, the work of producing a report for that month is minimal. The manager merely enters the data relating to that month and prints out the finished report. In

Exhibit 4-4 Summary Sheet

ACCOUNT:
PERIOD:

HOSPITAL OPERATIONS
VARIANCE ANALYSIS
FOR FISCAL 1983

EXPENSE CLASS	Y.T.D. BUDGET	Y.T.D. EXPENSE	$ VARIANCE	% VARIANCE	MONTHLY BUDGET	MONTHLY EXPENSE	$ VARIANCE	% VARIANCE
PROF. & ADMIN.	12654	11874	780	6.16	2109	2004	105	4.98
AFSCME	26431	27864	-1433	-5.42	4405	4233	172	3.91
OFFICE/CLERICAL	8312	7987	325	3.91	1385	1242	143	10.35
BENEFITS	4512	4312	200	4.43	752	877	-125	-16.62
OTHER PAYROLL	1576	1123	453	28.74	263	325	-62	-23.73
MEDICAL/SURGICAL	43984	48975	-4991	-11.35	7331	7222	109	1.48
GENERAL/OFFICE	12084	9086	2998	24.81	2014	1987	27	1.34
LAUNDRY	26432	22415	4017	15.20	4405	4215	190	4.32
PHARMACY	35421	34214	1207	3.41	5904	5618	286	4.84
POSTAGE	415	650	-235	-56.63	69	41	28	40.72
CONTRACT SERVICE	3654	4123	-469	-12.84	609	654	-45	-7.39
TELEPHONE	2643	2145	498	18.84	441	401	40	8.97
FOOD	314	200	114	36.31	52	44	8	15.92
EQUIPMENT DEPREC.	543	543	0	0.00	91	91	0	0.00
INTEREST EXPENSE	1163	1163	0	0.00	194	194	0	0.00
ACCOUNT TOTAL	180138	176674	3464	56	30023	29148	876	49
MATCHING FUNDS	1706	1706	0	0	284	285	0	0
TOTAL	178432	174968	3464	56	29739	28863	876	49

Exhibit 4-5 Expanded Summary Sheet: Patient Days

ACCOUNT:
PERIOD:

HOSPITAL OPERATION
VARIANCE ANALYSIS
ADJUSTED FOR PATIENT DAYS
FOR FISCAL 1983

EXPENSE CLASS	ADJ. Y.T.D. BUDGET	Y.T.D. EXPENSE	$ VARIANCE	% VARIANCE	ADJ. MONTHLY BUDGET	MONTHLY EXPENSE	$ VARIANCE	% VARIANCE
PROF. & ADMIN.	11864	11874	-10	-0.09	1907	2004	-97	-5.10
AFSCME	24780	27864	-3084	-12.45	3983	4233	-250	-6.28
OFFICE/CLERICAL	7793	7987	-194	-2.49	1252	1242	10	0.84
BENEFITS	4230	4312	-82	-1.93	680	877	-197	-28.99
OTHER PAYROLL	1478	1123	355	24.00	237	325	-88	-36.85
MEDICAL/SURGICAL	41237	48975	-7738	-18.77	6628	7222	-594	-8.97
GENERAL/OFFICE	11329	9086	2243	19.80	1821	1987	-166	-9.12
LAUNDRY	24781	22415	2366	9.55	3983	4215	-232	-5.83
PHARMACY	33208	34214	-1006	-3.03	5337	5618	-281	-5.26
POSTAGE	389	650	-261	-67.06	63	41	22	34.43
CONTRACT SERVICE	3426	4123	-697	-20.35	551	654	-103	-18.78
TELEPHONE	2478	2145	333	13.43	398	401	-3	-0.69
FOOD	294	200	94	32.06	47	44	3	7.00
EQUIPMENT DEPREC.	543	543	0	0.00	91	91	0	0.00
INTEREST EXPENSE	1163	1163	0	0.00	194	194	00	0.00
ACCOUNT TOTAL	167286	174968	-7682	-4.59	26887	28863	-1976	-7.35
MATCHING FUNDS	1706	1706	0	0.00	285	285	00	0.00
TOTAL	168992	176674	-7682	-4.55	27172	29148	-1976	-7.27

the case of the account summary illustrated above, the entire process takes about five minutes (including printing).

This particular report (Exhibit 4-4) was originally prepared by hand every month, taking about 45 minutes per account, plus about 20 minutes for typing. You can easily get an idea of the time saved by just one manager on one account. Consider the number of accounts over which specialized reports must be prepared—how many times have you rejected the idea of preparing a special report because of the time required to produce it?

UTILIZING SPREADSHEETS

From an administrative point of view, there are several ways of allocating the resource represented by spreadsheet programs. As we have discussed, the resource is so inexpensive that the administrator could allow everyone to "do his or her own thing" in preparing low level and summary reports. This can be useful, in that it allows people to contribute their own creative talents and specialized knowledge to the stream of information coming to the upper levels of the organization. The relatively small size of the program (in the case of VisiCalc) ensures limits to the scope and activity; that is, individuals cannot go too far afield on their own.

It is not always desirable to have a wide range of different formats. Often it is beneficial to utilize a more controlled, top-down approach in making use of this resource. After a suitable period of experimentation, the format of a report can be set for a period of time, with various levels of the report made available to appropriate persons.

In many organizations, a considerable degree of computerization already exists; it may not be necessary to duplicate data bases or reproduce reports for all account items. The items contributing to an administrative level cost summary might be shown as follows, along with their respective sources:

Expense Item	Source	Contribution	Reason
Linen	Dept. Supr.	DB; Cost rept.	Usage up-why
Med/Surg	Central DB	Bottom Line	Adeqate as is
Office	Dept. Supr.	DB; Cost rept.	Over budget
Pharmacy	Central DB	Bottom Line	Uses Pharmacy computer DB

It is quite useful in large organizations to have the small computer available as a source of analytic backup or in cases where the accuracy of data provided by another department or outside source is in doubt. Central data systems are typically unable to handle special requests for narrow-focus reports on a short-term basis; the micro provides them easily, once the requirements for the data base are met.

As we have seen, spreadsheet programs provide an excellent example of a stand-alone use of microcomputers. For many managers these programs may be the sole reason for purchasing a microcomputer. The environment allows the person with no formal computer training to implement problem-solving solutions using the machine. Obviously, there is a point at which the size of the spreadsheet, or the effort required to manage the associated data collection, becomes a limiting factor for the manager. If a manager begins a program on a small scale and then desires to expand in a large way, it is wise to consult with the appropriate data processing staff or information center regarding the relative costs of accomplishing the desired result on a microcomputer as compared with the mainframe. Performing computing tasks at the local level on a small scale can provide an excellent, low-cost method of testing the feasibility of system ideas.

Another implication that spreadsheet programs may have for data processing lies in their capability to accept data from files downloaded, or transferred electronically, from a larger computer system. Users should consider carefully whether or not some type of communication with an existing mainframe will become likely in the future. If the user has applications in mind that are known to require or involve the use of a mainframe data base, the data processing department must play an important role in the choice of the system. Although the task of accessing the data may seem simple, the casual user is not aware of the work that must be done to ensure that the microcomputer and the central mainframe computer can "talk" to each other effectively.

In smaller organizations or in individual departments, this kind of computerized report generation may not be present at all; the micros can make a real contribution to cost-effective use of resources with a relatively small expenditure. It only takes a few minutes of use to show even the most skeptical administrator why VisiCalc, for example, is the biggest-selling software program in the history of computer science. The flexibility of the operating environment will provide an outlet for many of the creative ideas relating to computers that seemed out of reach because of a lack of familiarity with mainframe systems.

Spreadsheet programs are indeed useful at every level of hospital management. The hospital supervisor can employ the program to track use of such things as individual supplies on a unit. The manager can make use of the detailed information provided at the supervisory level by treating it as a data base for analysis. Reports can easily be prepared comparing, say, budget versus expense or budgeted versus actual activity. At the administrator's level, the material reviewed might typically consist of account summaries and aggregate information regarding various aspects of hospitalwide activity or finance.

The manager, using the appropriate level of detail, is able to identify likely areas of concern to the administrator as well as respond to questions, often by assigning one or more supervisors the task of analyzing information in detail for single significant areas. Ideally, a well-maintained data base will aid in anticipating questions and be able to provide analyses more efficiently and effectively.

The supervisor is able to collect and analyze data on specific details such as supply or labor usage related to activity levels of any service. Information can be tracked over periods of time to show changes in activity or expenditures, for example.

Information, then, can flow from lower organizational levels to higher ones and be folded into the reports of managers at every level. The following applications illustrate the use of electronic spreadsheets by a number of departments as well as all administrative levels.

FACILITIES DATA BASE MANAGEMENT

The objective of this section is to present a number of useful spreadsheets to help deal with the responsibilities of facilities management. These spreadsheets were developed primarily for use by either a small hospital or a larger institution that can be conveniently subdivided into individual buildings or areas.

There are many uses for spreadsheet programs in facilities management. One simple spreadsheet is seen in Exhibit 4-6, which shows a cost summary for heating expenses in a facility. The monthly unit cost is used to show the price paid for electricity or gas in that period; the charge often changes month by month. Also, the number of days in the period is given; utilities often vary the number of days in the charge period from 25 to 35, which has its effect on cost for that period.

Exhibit 4-7 shows a hospital work order status sheet; it also includes a current charge for each work order (if available). The columns are fairly self-explanatory. The proposed completion date combined with the date of actual completion (and the run date) provide an accurate picture of the number of projects in an account that are being completed in a timely manner.

Exhibit 4-6 Cost Summary: Heating Expenses

HOSPITAL OPERATIONS RUN DATE: 07/01/83
FACILITY HEATING COSTS REVISED: 07/01/83
BUILDING: GENERAL HOSPITAL

DATE	METER READING	UNITS USED	MONTHLY COST	UNIT COST	DAYS IN PERIOD
6/30/83	4163				
7/30/83	4563	400	2433	6.08	31
8/29/83	4921	358	2166	6.05	30
9/30/83	5342	421	2675	6.35	32
10/29/83	5832	490	3299	6.73	30
11/30/83	6287	455	3217	7.07	32
12/30/83	6801	514	3899	7.59	31
1/29/83	7421	620	4325	6.98	30
2/28/83	8004	583	4102	7.04	29
3/27/83	8632	628	4475	7.13	27
4/30/83	9043	411	3014	7.33	32
5/30/83	9432	389	2589	6.66	31
6/29/83	9713	281	1789	6.37	30
TOTAL (OR AVG)		5550	37983	6.84	365

Exhibit 4-7 Hospital Work Order Status Sheet

HOSPITAL OPERATIONS
FACILITY: GENERAL HOSPITAL
ACCOUNT: 10101
ACCOUNT NAME: ADMINISTRATION
PERIOD: 07/01/83 TO 03/01/83

REVISED: 3/21/83
RUN DATE: 3/21/83

HWO #	SUBMITTED ON	WRITTEN BY	DESCRIPTION	TARGET DATE	% COMPL. AT RUN	ACTUAL COMPLETE	INCURRED EXPENSE
978823	08/21/82	W. CHRISTENSEN	REPLACE LOCK HARDWARE 1421	11/01/82	100	11/10/82	498.23
979988	09/15/82	W. CHRISTENSEN	INSTALL IPU CABINET	12/01/82	100	12/01/82	234.01
986653	11/01/82	E. STEARNS	PATCH AND PAINT SEC. SPACE	1/01/83	95		692.00
987543	12/07/82	W. CHRISTENSEN	PROVIDE NEW DOOR TO 1405	1/12/83	0		0.00
987312	12/18/82	W. CHRISTENSEN	INSTALL MARKER BOARD 4215	3/10/83	25		165.00
987345	1/10/83	E. STEARNS	INSTALL NEW EQUIPMENT 3156	2/11/83	50		1253.10
987152	1/03/83	W. CHRISTENSEN	MOVE EQUIPMENT FROM 1253 TO 5316	1/26/83	100	2/21/83	3516.43
987266	1/16/83	W. CHRISTENSEN	PATCH AND PAINT IPU ROOMS	4/01/83	30		417.50
987901	2/04/83	E. STEARNS	MODIFY 6109 FOR COMPUTER EQUIPMENT	5/20/83	0		0.00
					ACCOUNT TOTAL		6776.27

Exhibit 4-8 illustrates a simple space survey program. Although spreadsheet programs have only a limited utility in data base management, this program could serve as an informational resource for the number of square feet devoted to particular functions in the hospital. Note that the rooms are divided into a relatively small number of categories with the total square footage for each category given at the bottom of the sheet. Also, the percent of total square feet in the area is given for each category.

Figure 4-1 shows a simple use of the VisiTrend/VisiPlot graphics program presenting the information gathered on square footage associated with different kinds of room space. The graph illustrates in the pie chart format the distribution of space in the defined area.

The limitations of this kind of spreadsheet are obvious; with most programs it is not possible to sort even the information on the one sheet to give a list of all the patient rooms (for example). Also, most hospitals

---

Exhibit 4-8 Simple Space Survey Program

HOSPITAL OPERATIONS
FACILITY SPACE SURVEY
BUILDING: GENERAL HOSPITAL
AREA: 3 EAST

ROOM NUMBER	DESCRIPTION	SQ. FT. PT. ROOM	SQ. FT. OFFICE	SQ. FT. UTILITY	SQ. FT. PUBLIC	SQ. FT. BATH	SQ. FT. EXAM
3154	IPU SEMI PRIVATE	187					
3156	IPU SEMI PRIVATE	187					
3158	IPU SEMI PRIVATE	187					
3160	IPU SEMI PRIVATE	187					
3162	HEAD NURSE OFFICE		125				
3164	CLEAN STORAGE			110			
3166	NURSING STATION		210				
3168	IPU WAITING ROOM				140		
3170	IPU EXAM ROOM						145
3172	SOILED UTILITY			89			
3174	SOILED HOLDING			110			
3176	NURSE LOCKER ROOM		155				
3178T	PUBLIC TOILET					108	
3180	PATIENT BATH					79	
3181	IPU SEMI PRIVATE	195					
3183	IPU SEMI PRIVATE	195					
3185	IPU SEMI PRIVATE	195					
	TOTALS	585	490	309	140	187	145
	% OF TOTAL SQ. FT.	31.52	26.40	16.65	7.54	10.08	7.81

TOTAL SQUARE FEET: 1856

Figure 4-1 Distribution of Space: Pie Chart

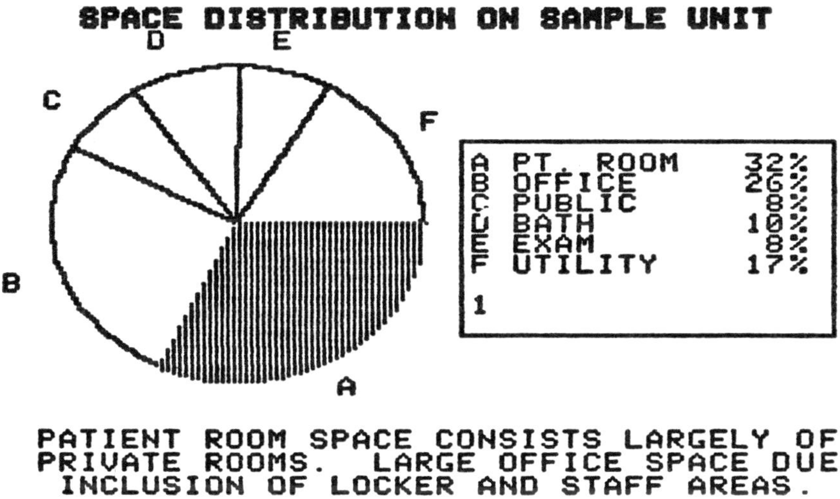

---

would require more than one sheet; as we have seen, separate spreadsheets do not usually "talk" to each other very well. Nevertheless, this program has a definite usefulness for space management at a very small price in setup cost and maintenance.

MATERIEL MANAGEMENT

Spreadsheet programs provide an ideal environment for limited use in materiel management. Depending on the size of the internal memory of the computer used (from 64K to 256K bytes), a fairly large amount of storage and manipulation can be performed.

The following examples will illustrate the use of spreadsheet programs to maintain a data base and then prepare reports based upon that information.

Consider the following: suppose you wanted to take a fairly intensive view of the linen usage in a particular unit or department. The first step would be to take the available data on the situation and place it in the machine in a simple tabular format. Exhibit 4-9 shows a three-year data base for linen expenses on a particular unit, with the individual usage

Exhibit 4-9 Data Base: Linen Usage

HOSPITAL OPERATIONS
LINEN USAGE FOR FISCAL 1978-79
FOR ACCOUNT 234567

RUN DATE: 02/05/83
REVISED: 02/05/83

LINEN USAGE FOR FISCAL 1980-81			COST	JULY	AUG	SEPT	OCT	NOV	DEC	YTD TOTAL	JAN	FEB	MAR	APRL	MAY	JUNE	ANN TOTAL
LINEN BAGS	9010105	EACH	0.20	200	198	210	194	189	114	1105	208	250	220	230	230	200	2443
BATHROBES	9010257	EACH	0.19	40	48	44	48	90	12	282	16	53	75	45	70	55	596
BATH BLANKETS	9010658	EACH	0.25	220	226	240	260	360	200	1506	340	350	300	310	270	190	3266
CLEANING CLOTHS		LB.	0.20	21	18	20	10	10	20	99	0	0	10	0	0	10	119
PATIENT GOWNS	9012059	EACH	0.21	120	110	110	40	110	30	520	45	165	120	120	150	125	1245
PAJAMA TOPS	9012503	EACH	0.09	230	260	260	270	440	140	1600	250	380	624	424	370	295	3943
PAJAMA BOTTOMS	9012606	EACH	0.09	230	260	260	240	410	140	1540	250	380	624	424	395	295	3908
PILLOW CASES	9012953	EACH	0.06	700	670	720	600	850	400	3940	680	800	720	980	800	760	8680
LARGE SHEETS	9013209	EACH	0.29	898	910	940	840	970	420	4978	920	1000	900	1000	1000	900	10698
BED SPREADS	9014706	EACH	0.48	145	140	165	130	210	100	890	160	175	120	160	175	130	1810
SOCKS	9014408	EACH	0.01	200	190	210	180	318	105	1203	140	270	620	280	180	100	2793
BATH TOWELS	9014901	EACH	0.09	1190	1200	1210	840	1310	490	6240	870	1100	1270	1400	1050	1000	12930
WASH CLOTHS	9015450	EACH	0.16	1090	1130	1110	840	1130	490	5790	830	1100	1200	1300	1050	1000	12270

LINEN USAGE FOR FISCAL 1981-82			COST	JULY	AUG	SEPT	OCT	NOV	DEC	YTD TOTAL	JAN	FEB	MAR	APRL	MAY	JUNE	ANN TOTAL
LINEN BAGS	9010105	EACH	0.23	220	200	200	180	270	170	1240	200	210	200	220	210	240	2520
BATHROBES	9010257	EACH	0.22	45	75	75	50	65	40	350	55	105	120	115	45	45	835
BATH BLANKETS	9010658	EACH	0.29	200	160	200	190	280	180	1210	250	230	180	220	180	220	2490
CLEANING CLOTHS		LB.	0.23	30	10	20	20	0	30	110	20	10	20	10	10	10	190
PATIENT GOWNS	9012059	EACH	0.28	125	170	155	115	170	135	870	105	75	100	100	70	100	1420
PAJAMA TOPS	9012503	EACH	0.11	345	395	370	280	345	230	1965	515	635	720	510	205	270	4820

PAJAMA BOTTOMS	9012606	EACH	0.11	345	425	360	280	335	190	1935	365	516	615	510	205	270	4416
PILLOW CASES	9012753	EACH	0.07	560	640	720	480	800	480	3680	640	600	650	720	520	700	7510
LARGE SHEETS	9013209	EACH	0.34	700	800	800	600	900	600	4400	800	810	770	880	640	900	9200
BED SPREADS	9014706	EACH	0.56	135	135	145	125	185	110	835	90	110	130	135	95	150	1545
SOCKS	9014408	EACH	0.02	200	180	220	190	185	110	1085	295	278	510	340	120	180	2808
BATH TOWELS	9014901	EACH	0.11	950	900	1050	850	1100	800	5650	1000	1200	1200	1300	750	1200	12300
WASH CLOTHS	9015450	EACH	0.01	1030	1000	1100	850	1100	800	5880	1050	1200	1100	1300	750	1200	12480

LINEN USAGE FOR FISCAL 1982-83			COST	JULY	AUG	SEPT	OCT	NOV	DEC	YTD TOTAL	JAN	FEB	MAR	APRL	MAY	JUNE	ANN TOTAL
LINEN BAGS	9010105	EACH	0.37	190	160	240	180	160	200	1130	160	180	0	0	0	0	1470
BATHROBES	9010257	EACH	0.36	60	46	50	55	45	40	296	40	55	0	0	0	0	391
BATH BLANKETS	9010658	EACH	0.48	140	220	300	260	210	250	1380	280	230	0	0	0	0	1890
CLEANING CLOTHS		LB.	0.37	0	10	10	10	0	10	40	20	10	0	0	0	0	70
PATIENT GOWNS	9012059	EACH	0.45	90	120	170	140	110	80	710	80	90	0	0	0	0	880
PAJAMA TOPS	9012503	EACH	0.17	236	225	300	330	270	305	1666	3355	300	0	0	0	0	5321
PAJAMA BOTTOMS	9012606	EACH	0.17	250	200	340	330	270	305	1695	320	300	0	0	0	0	2315
PILLOW CASES	9012953	EACH	0.11	680	730	940	760	620	660	4390	630	580	0	0	0	0	5600
LARGE SHEETS	9013209	EACH	0.56	850	850	1170	950	840	830	5490	810	800	0	0	0	0	7100
BED SPREADS	9014706	EACH	0.91	140	150	205	155	120	130	900	130	135	0	0	0	0	1165
SOCKS	9014408	EACH	0.02	120	110	140	160	160	180	870	190	220	0	0	0	0	1280
BATH TOWELS	9014901	EACH	0.17	1050	1050	1300	1000	850	800	6050	900	950	0	0	0	0	7900
WASH CLOTHS	9015450	EACH	0.02	1050	1100	1400	1050	850	800	6250	900	900	0	0	0	0	8050

figures included on a monthly basis. Totals have been added at the end of the year indicating annual usage per item.

These data are typed in exactly as shown in Exhibit 4-9; the only formulas entered calculate the totals necessary. An obvious benefit is that the data base is present in one simple and easily readable format. The particular advantage of having it on the computer is that we can now prepare reports based on this information, with a significant saving in preparation time.

Remember that the spreadsheet can be divided into areas that can be printed out as separate sheets later. Suppose, for example, that you wanted to have a cost accounting of the linen usage, as in Exhibit 4-9. Finding the monthly cost for each item is done by multiplying the number of items used by the cost per item. Rather than retype all of the usage figures, why not set up another table "below" the one established for linen usage?

Exhibit 4-10 illustrates a report set up in a manner similar to that used in the linen usage report introduced earlier. Note that the actual prices for each linen item are included in the second column. This report differs from the first linen report in that all of the expense figures are derived directly from the usage report.

The dollar amount spent on each item per month is defined by multiplying the contents of the cell containing the price of that item by the contents of the cell containing the number of items used that month.

Another useful report is an accounting of the number of items used per patient day in any given month. One could, of course, provide a report detailing the expense per patient day; however, a comparison of expense from one year to the next may not yield useful information on the "actual" dollars expended (owing to inflationary increases, price increases)—more on this aspect later.

In order to produce this report, it is necessary to add some information to our data base; namely, the number of patient days on this unit for the months covered by the report. This may be done by appending this information to the bottom of the usage report (see Exhibit 4-11); this information may be left out when producing the usage report by carefully defining the area to be printed.

The new report is prepared in the same way as the linen expense report; the number of pieces of linen per patient day for each month is arrived at by dividing the contents of the cell containing the number of pieces by the contents of the cell containing the number of patient days. The resulting report is shown in Exhibit 4-12.

When saving this report for disk storage, it is not necessary to save the original data base over and over again. A more efficient storage method is to create your report based on the original usage figures and then blank

Exhibit 4-10 Expanded Usage Report: Linen Costs

HOSPITAL OPERATIONS
LINEN COST FOR FISCAL 1980-83
FOR ACCOUNT 234567

LINEN COST FOR FISCAL 1981			COST	JULY	AUG	SEPT	OCT	NOV	DEC	TOTAL	JAN	FEB	MAR	APRL	MAY	JUNE	TOTAL
LINEN BAGS	9010105	EACH	0.20	40	40	42	39	38	23	221	42	50	44	46	46	40	489
BATHROBES	9010257	EACH	0.19	8	9	8	9	17	2	54	3	10	14	9	13	10	113
BATH BLANKETS	9010658	EACH	0.25	55	57	60	65	90	50	377	85	88	75	78	68	48	817
CLEANING CLOTHS		LB.	0.20	4	4	4	2	2	4	20	0	0	2	0	0	2	24
PATIENT GOWNS	9012059	EACH	0.21	25	23	23	8	23	6	109	9	35	25	25	32	26	261
PAJAMA TOPS	9012503	EACH	0.09	21	23	23	24	40	13	144	23	34	56	38	33	27	355
PAJAMA BOTTOMS	9012606	EACH	0.09	21	23	23	22	37	13	139	23	34	56	38	36	27	352
PILLOW CASES	9012953	EACH	0.06	42	40	43	36	51	24	236	41	48	43	59	48	46	521
LARGE SHEETS	9013209	EACH	0.29	260	264	273	244	281	122	1444	267	290	261	290	290	261	3102
BED SPREADS	9014706	EACH	0.48	70	67	79	62	101	48	427	77	84	58	77	84	62	869
SOCKS	9014408	EACH	0.01	2	2	2	2	3	1	12	1	3	6	3	2	1	28
BATH TOWELS	9014901	EACH	0.09	107	108	109	76	118	44	562	78	99	114	126	95	90	1164
WASH CLOTHS	9015450	EACH	0.02	17	18	18	13	18	8	93	13	18	19	21	17	16	196
	TOTALS			672	678	708	602	819	357	3836	661	792	774	809	762	655	8290

LINEN USAGE FOR FISCAL 1982			COST	JULY	AUG	SEPT	OCT	NOV	DEC	TOTAL	JAN	FEB	MAR	APRL	MAY	JUNE	TOTAL
LINEN BAGS	9010105	EACH	0.23	51	46	46	41	62	39	285	46	48	46	51	48	55	580
BATHROBES	9010257	EACH	0.22	10	17	17	11	14	9	77	12	10	26	25	10	10	184
BATH BLANKETS	9010658	EACH	0.29	58	46	58	55	81	52	351	73	88	52	64	52	64	722
CLEANING CLOTHS		LB.	0.23	7	2	5	5	0	7	25	5	0	5	2	2	2	44
PATIENT GOWNS	9012059	EACH	0.28	35	48	43	32	48	38	244	29	35	28	28	20	28	398
PAJAMA TOPS	9012503	EACH	0.11	38	43	41	31	38	25	216	57	34	79	56	23	30	530
PAJAMA BOTTOMS	9012606	EACH	0.11	38	47	40	31	37	21	213	40	34	68	56	23	30	486

Exhibit 4-10 continued

LINEN COST FOR FISCAL 1981			COST	JULY	AUG	SEPT	OCT	NOV	DEC	TOTAL	JAN	FEB	MAR	APRL	MAY	JUNE	TOTAL
PILLOW CASES	9012953	EACH	0.07	39	45	50	34	56	34	258	45	48	46	50	36	49	526
LARGE SHEETS	9013209	EACH	0.34	238	272	272	204	306	204	1496	272	290	262	299	218	306	3128
BED SPREADS	9014706	EACH	0.56	76	76	81	70	104	62	468	50	84	73	76	53	84	865
SOCKS	9014408	EACH	0.02	4	4	4	4	4	2	22	6	3	10	7	2	4	56
BATH TOWELS	9014901	EACH	0.11	105	99	116	94	121	88	622	110	99	132	143	83	132	1353
WASH CLOTHS	9015450	EACH	0.01	10	10	11	9	11	8	59	11	18	11	13	8	12	125
	TOTALS			708	754	783	619	881	588	4334	755	790	837	870	577	805	8996

LINEN USAGE FOR FISCAL 1983			COST	JULY	AUG	SEPT	OCT	NOV	DEC	TOTAL	JAN	FEB	MAR	APRL	MAY	JUNE	TOTAL
LINEN BAGS	9010105	EACH	0.37	70	59	89	67	59	74	418	59	67	0	0	0	0	544
BATHROBES	9010257	EACH	0.36	22	17	18	20	16	14	107	14	20	0	0	0	0	141
BATH BLANKETS	9010658	EACH	0.48	67	106	144	125	101	120	662	134	110	0	0	0	0	907
CLEANING CLOTHS		LB.	0.37	0	4	4	4	0	4	15	7	4	0	0	0	0	26
PATIENT GOWNS	9012059	EACH	0.45	41	54	77	63	50	36	320	36	41	0	0	0	0	396
PAJAMA TOPS	9012503	EACH	0.17	40	38	51	56	46	52	283	570	51	0	0	0	0	905
PAJAMA BOTTOMS	9012606	EACH	0.17	43	34	58	56	46	52	288	54	51	0	0	0	0	394
PILLOW CASES	9012953	EACH	0.11	75	80	103	84	68	73	483	69	64	0	0	0	0	616
LARGE SHEETS	9013209	EACH	0.56	476	476	655	532	470	465	3074	454	448	0	0	0	0	3976
BED SPREADS	9014706	EACH	0.91	127	137	187	141	109	118	819	118	123	0	0	0	0	1060
SOCKS	901440C	EACH	0.02	2	2	3	3	3	4	17	4	4	0	0	0	0	26
BATH TOWELS	9014901	EACH	0.17	179	179	221	170	145	136	1029	153	162	0	0	0	0	1343
WASH CLOTHS	9015450	EACH	0.02	21	22	28	21	17	16	125	18	18	0	0	0	0	161
	TOTALS			1162	1207	1637	1341	1130	1163	7640	1692	1162	0	0	0	0	10494

Exhibit 4-11 Expanded Usage Report: Patient Days

HOSPITAL OPERATIONS
LINEN USAGE FOR FISCAL 1978-79
FOR ACCOUNT 234567

RUN DATE: 02/05/83
REVISED: 02/05/83

LINEN USAGE FOR FISCAL 1980-81			COST	JULY	AUG	SEPT	OCT	NOV	DEC	YTD TOTAL	JAN	FEB	MAR	APRL	MAY	JUNE	ANN TOTAL
LINEN BAGS	9010105	EACH	0.20	200	198	210	194	189	114	1105	208	250	220	230	230	200	2443
BATHROBES	9010257	EACH	0.19	40	48	44	48	90	12	282	16	53	75	45	70	55	596
BATH BLANKETS	9010658	EACH	0.25	220	226	240	260	360	200	1506	340	350	300	310	270	190	3266
CLEANING CLOTHS		LB.	0.20	21	18	20	10	10	20	99	0	0	10	0	0	10	119
PATIENT GOWNS	9012059	EACH	0.21	120	110	110	40	110	30	520	45	165	120	120	150	125	1245
PAJAMA TOPS	9012503	EACH	0.09	230	260	260	270	440	140	1600	250	380	624	424	370	295	3943
PAJAMA BOTTOMS	9012606	EACH	0.09	230	260	260	240	410	140	1540	250	380	624	424	395	295	3908
PILLOW CASES	9012953	EACH	0.06	700	670	720	600	850	400	3940	680	800	720	980	800	760	8680
LARGE SHEETS	9013209	EACH	0.29	898	910	940	840	970	420	4978	920	1000	900	1000	1000	900	10698
BED SPREADS	9014706	EACH	0.48	145	140	165	130	210	100	890	160	175	120	160	175	130	1810
SOCKS	9014408	EACH	0.01	200	190	210	180	318	105	1203	140	270	620	280	180	100	2793
BATH TOWELS	9014901	EACH	0.09	1190	1200	1210	840	1310	490	6240	870	1100	1270	1400	1050	1000	12930
WASH CLOTHS	9015450	EACH	0.16	1090	1130	1110	840	1130	490	5790	830	1100	1200	1300	1050	1000	12270
			PT DAY	566	580	616	544	652	333	3291	625	633	629	705	579	630	7092
			ADMITS	138	141	150	133	159	81	803	152	154	153	172	141	154	1730

LINEN USAGE FOR FISCAL 1981-82			COST	JULY	AUG	SEPT	OCT	NOV	DEC	YTD TOTAL	JAN	FEB	MAR	APRL	MAY	JUNE	ANN TOTAL
LINEN BAGS	9010105	EACH	0.23	220	200	200	180	270	170	1240	200	210	200	220	210	240	2520
BATHROBES	9010257	EACH	0.22	45	75	75	50	65	40	350	55	105	120	115	45	45	835
BATH BLANKETS	9010658	EACH	0.29	200	160	200	190	280	180	1210	250	230	180	220	180	220	2490
CLEANING CLOTHS		LB.	0.23	30	10	20	20	0	30	110	20	10	20	10	10	10	190
PATIENT GOWNS	9012059	EACH	0.28	125	170	155	115	170	135	870	105	75	100	100	70	100	1420
PAJAMA TOPS	9012503	EACH	0.11	345	395	370	280	345	230	1965	515	635	720	510	205	270	4820

Exhibit 4-11 continued

LINEN USAGE FOR FISCAL 1980-81			COST	JULY	AUG	SEPT	OCT	NOV	DEC	YTD TOTAL	JAN	FEB	MAR	APRL	MAY	JUNE	ANN TOTAL
PAJAMA BOTTOMS	9012606	EACH	0.11	345	425	360	280	335	190	1935	365	516	615	510	205	270	4416
PILLOW CASES	9012953	EACH	0.07	560	640	720	480	800	480	3680	640	600	650	720	520	700	7510
LARGE SHEETS	9013209	EACH	0.34	700	800	800	600	900	600	4400	800	810	770	880	640	900	9200
BED SPREADS	9014706	EACH	0.56	135	135	145	125	185	110	835	90	110	130	135	95	150	1545
SOCKS	9014408	EACH	0.02	200	180	220	190	185	110	1085	295	278	510	340	120	180	2808
BATH TOWELS	9014901	EACH	0.11	950	900	1050	850	1100	800	5650	1000	1200	1200	1300	750	1200	12300
WASH CLOTHS	9015450	EACH	0.01	1030	1000	1100	850	1100	800	5880	1050	1200	1100	1300	750	1200	12480
			PT DAY	556	621	536	545	514	361	3133	589	554	584	646	485	598	6589
			ADMITS	121	135	117	118	112	78	681	128	120	127	140	105	130	1432

LINEN USAGE FOR FISCAL 1982-83			COST	JULY	AUG	SEPT	OCT	NOV	DEC	YTD TOTAL	JAN	FEB	MAR	APRL	MAY	JUNE	ANN TOTAL
LINEN BAGS	9010105	EACH	0.37	190	160	240	180	160	200	1130	160	180	0	0	0	0	1470
BATHROBES	9010257	EACH	0.36	60	46	50	55	45	40	296	40	55	0	0	0	0	391
BATH BLANKETS	9010658	EACH	0.48	140	220	300	260	210	250	1380	280	230	0	0	0	0	1890
CLEANING CLOTHS		LB.	0.37	0	10	10	10	0	10	40	20	10	0	0	0	0	70
PATIENT GOWNS	9012059	EACH	0.45	90	120	170	140	110	80	710	80	90	0	0	0	0	880
PAJAMA TOPS	9012503	EACH	0.17	236	225	300	330	270	305	1666	3355	300	0	0	0	0	5321
PAJAMA BOTTOMS	9012606	EACH	0.17	250	200	340	330	270	305	1695	320	300	0	0	0	0	2315
PILLOW CASES	9012953	EACH	0.11	680	730	940	760	620	660	4390	630	580	0	0	0	0	5600
LARGE SHEETS	9013209	EACH	0.56	850	850	1170	950	840	830	5490	810	800	0	0	0	0	7100
BED SPREADS	9014706	EACH	0.91	140	150	205	155	120	130	900	130	135	0	0	0	0	1165
SOCKS	9014408	EACH	0.02	120	110	140	160	160	180	870	190	220	0	0	0	0	1280
BATH TOWELS	9014901	EACH	0.17	1050	1050	1300	1000	850	800	6050	900	950	0	0	0	0	7900
WASH CLOTHS	9015450	EACH	0.02	1050	1100	1400	1050	850	800	6250	900	900	0	0	0	0	8050
			PT DAY	617	621	660	690	527	422	3537	512	452	0	0	0	0	4501
			ADMITS	147	148	157	164	125	100	842	122	108	0	0	0	0	1072

Exhibit 4-12 Expanded Usage Report: Linen Use Per Patient Day

HOSPITAL OPERATIONS
LINEN USE/PT DAY FOR FISCAL 1981-83
FOR ACCOUNT 10606

LINEN USE PER PT. DAY FY81			UNIT COST	U/PD JULY	U/PD AUG	U/PD SEPT	U/PD OCT	U/PD NOV	U/PD DEC	YTD AVG	U/PD JAN	U/PD FEB	U/PD MAR	U/PD APRL	U/PD MAY	U/PD JUNE	ANN AVG
LINEN BAGS	9010105	EACH	0.20	0.35	0.34	0.34	0.36	0.29	0.34	0.34	0.33	0.39	0.35	0.33	0.40	0.32	0.34
BATHROBES	9010257	EACH	0.19	0.07	0.08	0.08	0.09	0.14	0.04	0.09	0.03	0.08	0.12	0.06	0.12	0.09	0.08
BATH BLANKETS	9010658	EACH	0.25	0.39	0.39	0.44	0.48	0.55	0.60	0.46	0.54	0.55	0.48	0.44	0.47	0.30	0.46
CLEANING CLOTHS		LB.	0.20	0.04	0.03	0.04	0.02	0.02	0.06	0.03	0.00	0.00	0.02	0.00	0.00	0.02	0.02
PATIENT GOWNS	9012059	EACH	0.21	0.21	0.19	0.20	0.07	0.17	0.09	0.16	0.07	0.26	0.19	0.17	0.26	0.20	0.18
PAJAMA TOPS	9012503	EACH	0.09	0.41	0.45	0.48	0.50	0.67	0.42	0.49	0.40	0.60	0.99	0.60	0.64	0.47	0.56
PAJAMA BOTTOMS	9012606	EACH	0.09	0.41	0.45	0.48	0.44	0.63	0.42	0.47	0.40	0.60	0.99	0.60	0.68	0.47	0.55
PILLOW CASES	9012953	EACH	0.06	1.24	1.16	1.32	1.10	1.30	1.20	1.20	1.09	1.26	1.14	1.39	1.38	1.21	1.22
LARGE SHEETS	9013209	EACH	0.29	1.59	1.57	1.73	1.54	1.49	1.26	1.51	1.47	1.58	1.43	1.42	1.73	1.43	1.51
BED SPREADS	9014706	EACH	0.48	0.26	0.24	0.30	0.24	0.32	0.30	0.27	0.26	0.28	0.19	0.23	0.30	0.21	0.26
SOCKS	9014408	EACH	0.01	0.35	0.33	0.39	0.33	0.49	0.32	0.37	0.22	0.43	0.99	0.40	0.31	0.16	0.39
BATH TOWELS	9014901	EACH	0.09	2.10	2.07	2.22	1.54	2.01	1.47	1.90	1.39	1.74	2.02	1.99	1.81	1.59	1.82
WASH CLOTHS	9015450	EACH	0.01	1.93	1.95	2.04	1.54	1.73	1.47	1.76	1.33	1.74	1.91	1.84	1.81	1.59	1.73

LINEN USE PER PT. DAY FY82			UNIT COST	U/PD JULY	U/PD AUG	U/PD SEPT	U/PD OCT	U/PD NOV	U/PD DEC	YTD AVG	U/PD JAN	U/PD FEB	U/PD MAR	U/PD APRL	U/PD MAY	U/PD JUNE	ANN AVG
LINEN BAGS	9010105	EACH	0.23	0.40	0.32	0.37	0.33	0.53	0.47	0.40	0.34	0.38	0.34	0.34	0.43	0.40	0.38
BATHROBES	9010257	EACH	0.22	0.08	0.12	0.14	0.09	0.13	0.11	0.11	0.09	0.19	0.21	0.18	0.09	0.08	0.13
BATH BLANKETS	9010658	EACH	0.29	0.36	0.26	0.37	0.35	0.54	0.50	0.39	0.42	0.42	0.31	0.34	0.37	0.37	0.38
CLEANING CLOTHS	DAY FY	LB.	0.23	0.05	0.02	0.04	0.04	0.00	0.08	0.04	0.03	0.02	0.03	0.02	0.02	0.02	0.03

Exhibit 4-12 continued

LINEN USE PER PT. DAY FY81			UNIT COST	U/PD JULY	U/PD AUG	U/PD SEPT	U/PD OCT	U/PD NOV	U/PD DEC	YTD AVG	U/PD JAN	U/PD FEB	U/PD MAR	U/PD APRL	U/PD MAY	U/PD JUNE	ANN AVG
PATIENT GOWNS	9012059	EACH	0.28	0.22	0.27	0.29	0.21	0.33	0.37	0.28	0.18	0.14	0.17	0.15	0.14	0.17	0.22
PAJAMA TOPS	9012503	EACH	0.11	0.62	0.64	0.69	0.51	0.67	0.64	0.63	0.87	1.15	1.23	0.79	0.42	0.45	0.73
PAJAMA BOTTOMS	9012606	EACH	0.11	0.62	0.68	0.67	0.51	0.65	0.53	0.62	0.62	0.93	1.05	0.79	0.42	0.45	0.67
PILLOW CASES	9012953	EACH	0.07	1.01	1.03	1.34	0.88	1.56	1.33	1.17	1.09	1.08	1.11	1.11	1.07	1.17	1.14
LARGE SHEETS	9013209	EACH	0.34	1.26	1.29	1.49	1.10	1.75	1.66	1.40	1.36	1.46	1.32	1.36	1.32	1.50	1.40
BED SPREADS	9014706	EACH	0.56	0.24	0.22	0.27	0.23	0.36	0.30	0.27	0.15	0.20	0.22	0.21	0.20	0.25	0.23
SOCKS TOPS	9014408	EACH	0.02	0.36	0.29	0.41	0.35	0.36	0.30	0.35	0.50	0.50	0.87	0.53	0.25	0.30	0.43
BATH TOWELS	9014901	EACH	0.11	1.71	1.45	1.96	1.56	2.14	2.22	1.80	1.70	2.17	2.05	2.01	1.55	2.01	1.87
WASH CLOTHS	9015450	EACH	0.01	1.85	1.61	2.05	1.56	2.14	2.22	1.88	1.78	2.17	1.88	2.01	1.55	2.01	1.89

LINEN USE PER PT. DAY FOR FY83			UNIT COST	U/PD JULY	U/PD AUG	U/PD SEPT	U/PD OCT	U/PD NOV	U/PD DEC	YTD AVG	U/PD JAN	U/PD FEB	U/PD MAR	U/PD APRL	U/PD MAY	U/PD JUNE	YTD AVG
LINEN BAGS	9010105	EACH	0.37	0.31	0.26	0.36	0.26	0.30	0.47	0.32	0.31	0.40	0.00	0.00	0.00	0.00	0.33
BATHROBES	9010257	EACH	0.36	0.10	0.07	0.08	0.08	0.09	0.09	0.08	0.08	0.12	0.00	0.00	0.00	0.00	0.09
BATH BLANKETS	9010658	EACH	0.48	0.23	0.35	0.45	0.38	0.40	0.59	0.39	0.55	0.51	0.00	0.00	0.00	0.00	0.42
CLEANING CLOTHS	DAY FY	LB.	0.37	0.00	0.02	0.02	0.01	0.00	0.02	0.01	0.04	0.02	0.00	0.00	0.00	0.00	0.02
PATIENT GOWNS	9012059	EACH	0.45	0.15	0.19	0.26	0.20	0.21	0.19	0.20	0.16	0.20	0.00	0.00	0.00	0.00	0.20
PAJAMA TOPS	9012503	EACH	0.17	0.38	0.36	0.45	0.48	0.51	0.72	0.47	6.55	0.66	0.00	0.00	0.00	0.00	1.18
PAJAMA BOTTOMS	9012606	EACH	0.17	0.41	0.32	0.52	0.48	0.51	0.72	0.48	0.62	0.66	0.00	0.00	0.00	0.00	0.51
PILLOW CASES	9012953	EACH	0.11	1.10	1.18	1.42	1.10	1.18	1.56	1.24	1.23	1.28	0.00	0.00	0.00	0.00	1.24
LARGE SHEETS	9013209	EACH	0.56	1.38	1.37	1.77	1.38	1.59	1.97	1.55	1.58	1.77	0.00	0.00	0.00	0.00	1.58
BED SPREADS	9014706	EACH	0.91	0.23	0.24	0.31	0.22	0.23	0.31	0.25	0.25	0.30	0.00	0.00	0.00	0.00	0.26
SOCKS TOPS	9014408	EACH	0.02	0.19	0.18	0.21	0.23	0.30	0.43	0.25	0.37	0.49	0.00	0.00	0.00	0.00	0.28
BATH TOWELS	9014901	EACH	0.17	1.70	1.69	1.97	1.45	1.61	1.90	1.71	1.76	2.10	0.00	0.00	0.00	0.00	1.76
WASH CLOTHS	9015450	EACH	0.02	1.70	1.77	2.12	1.52	1.61	1.90	1.77	1.76	1.99	0.00	0.00	0.00	0.00	1.79

out the original figures, leaving only the new report. In the examples shown, the data base ranges from rows 1 through 55; the secondary reports range from 56 to 100. For the secondary reports, only rows 56 to 100 need be saved; this saves on disk storage space.

The information from these reports can then be folded into an administrative summary report with the minimum details needed to convey the findings of the manager based on the reports prepared.

Together, these programs provide a simple data base management approach for linen usage and cost. The level of detail provided is adequate at all levels of the organization, a situation not typically noted with reports produced by centralized data processing departments. Most centralized DP efforts are aimed at pleasing the higher levels of the organization.

The advantage to having this information on a microcomputer in this form is that the information can be easily manipulated on the unit level; the maximum in flexibility is provided to all levels of the organization, in terms of allowing each level of personnel to format reports for its own needs.

PRODUCTIVITY MEASUREMENT

The measurement of productivity in hospitals is and will continue to be a subject of high interest during the remainder of the 1980s. As pressures for cost containment and competition become greater—which they no doubt will because of the economic stresses faced by federal and state governments, industry, and financial institutions—hospitals will be forced to find ways to achieve greater productivity with existing resources or of maintaining productivity levels with reduced resources.

The purpose of this section is to suggest ways of utilizing a microcomputer to assist in productivity measurement. The user is encouraged to become as creative as possible, within the framework of his or her own organizational mission, policies, and economic constraints.

Types of Productivity Measurement

There are three types of productivity measurement with which a hospital may deal: total factor productivity, partial factor productivity, and simple outcome indicators.

Total factor productivity is the measure of ratios between total output to total input. Input includes labor, materials, energy, capital, and perhaps other factors. Its formula would be:

$$\frac{\text{Total Output}}{\text{Labor} + \text{Materials} + \text{Energy} + \text{Capital}}$$

Partial factor productivity measurement is used when the productivity of a single factor is wanted, such as total output related to labor input.

Outcome indicators may be useful in studies of satisfaction of patients or physicians. An example of such an indicator would be:

$$\frac{\text{Total Admissions}}{\text{Number of Complaints}}$$

The purpose of the measurement determines the type of measurement to be employed. Short-term labor productivity measurements might be employed when a hospital has a need to know, for example, the usefulness of certain production processes, the efficacy of certain services with respect to resource consumption, or the usefulness of a particular technology that is perceived to be cost saving. Partial factor productivity measurement might be quite useful in determining the usefulness of an institutional investment in physical productivity improvements. That is, the productivity of cash resources, which might be scarce, can be described in terms of the ability of those resources to produce investment income as compared with their ability to produce income (or reduce costs) if invested in physical improvements.

Physical Measurements

Physical measurements are measurements of things such as numbers of employees or labor hours worked to produce a given product or product element; they are also measurements of materials (supplies or equipment) used in production. Physical measurements will undoubtedly be a major focus of hospital productivity measurement systems because of the labor intensity of many hospital operations.

Financial Productivity

Financial productivity consists of the measurement of, for example, labor inputs in terms of wage or salary payments, fringe benefits, or nonproductive time. In physical terms, the quantity of labor required for production would be measured; in financial terms, measurement would involve labor costs per unit of output.

Electronic spreadsheet programs are useful tools for analyzing productivity (particularly on a small scale) by building data bases that span a period of time or allow for comparison of many large sets of numbers. These systems enable the user to establish predetermined standards for storage and comparison with data related to activity. Standards may also be derived by comparing activity and performance over many time periods, with indexes derived from the data. The VisiCalc program, for example, can measure productivity as a ratio of actual hours used to perform an activity or supply a service compared to the standard number of hours required to perform such an activity.

The spreadsheet allows the user to enter and update data and perform hundreds of repetitious calculations on a routine basis, in a fraction of the time required to do the same task manually. The time-saving value of this approach results from the reduced number of required data entry and calculation tasks once the desired model and formulas have been entered. Exhibit 4-13 is a simple example of a general purpose labor cost algorithm using a very small amount of data. The use of the index to measure changes over time closely demonstrates productivity changes.

This exhibit demonstrates in a simple way how numbers can be easily manipulated by a microcomputer using a spreadsheet program. The BASE

Exhibit 4-13 General Purpose Productivity Measurement: Labor Costs

	General	Base Period and Ratios	Indexes
	Base Period Amount	Currrent Amount	Current Index
Units	10,000	15,000	150.00%
Hours	1,000	1,400	140.00%
Payroll	$12,000.00	$19,600.00	163.33%
Pay/Hour	$12.00	$14.00	116.67%
Units/Hour	10.00	10.71	107.14%
Pay/Unit	$1.20	$1.31	108.89%

PERIOD AMOUNT column includes data that are entered by the user as well as data that are computed from the entered data. The PAY PER HOUR, UNITS PER HOUR, and PAY PER UNIT calculations are based on previously established formulas. The information in the last column, INDEX, is derived by entering a formula that divides the information in the first numerical column by that in the second. This formula is easily replicated throughout the entire last column by a simple method using only a few steps.

Once this has been done, it can be repeated for large numbers of lines of data. It is a feature that is available every time this particular model is used. Since this model represents the change in productivity for a specific task from a base period to a subsequent period, it is quite useful both as a presentation of a measure of productivity showing historically based standards and as an index. The index has the advantage of being able to calculate or convert to other indexes. It is also useful in plotting trends and in calculating percentages.

Housekeeping Productivity Model

Another example of simple electronic spreadsheet use (Exhibit 4-14) involves measuring housekeeping labor performance using actual hours required to clean various types of patient rooms compared with an established time standard. Here again, the formulas required to analyze and present this information are entered only once and are replicated as necessary throughout the model. In this model, the STANDARD HOURS earned is a function of the standard time required to clean each type of room multiplied by the number of such rooms cleaned. The actual hours are entered by the user, as is the actual quantity of rooms cleaned. The spreadsheet computes the INDEX as well as all ratios. In this example, the department is experiencing a negative variance by virtue of having used more hours than the established standard. The average time required to clean a room and the average number of rooms cleaned per hour are thus below standard. This information may be helpful to hospital management in analyzing reasons for expense budget variances, patient complaints, grievance traffic, and staffing requirements.

Such systems are quite useful to department heads in controlling labor use and in predicting and justifying labor needs. In conjunction with labor cost information that might be produced by the hospital's budget and expense reporting system, the department head can more accurately predict and control labor costs while maintaining adequate production and quality through such means as assignment or reassignment of staff and more judicious use of overtime. The electronic merging of the information,

Exhibit 4-14 Productivity Measurement: Housekeeping

PRODUCT MEASURES
BASED ON RATIOS OF ACTUAL TO STANDARD HOURS

HOUSEKEEPING
MAY, 1983

MEASURES	QUANTITY	STANDARD HOURS	ACTUAL HOURS	% PROD. STD=100
TOT. ROOMS CLEANED	2205			
STANDARD ROOMS	1145			
CUSTOM ROOMS	701			
DELUXE ROOMS	359			
BASIC HRS/RM STD	.5	572.5	545	105.05
CUSTOM HRS/RM STD	.1	70.1	95	73.79
DELUXE HRS/RM STD	.2	71.8	85	84.47
TOT. HRS		714.4	725	98.54

RATIOS	STANDARD	ACTUAL	PERCENT
AV CLEANING HRS/RM	0.32	0.33	101.48
ROOMS CLEANED/HR	3.09	3.04	101.48

even into a simple spreadsheet format, could produce a powerful tool in the hands of an astute department head.

Social Work Productivity Model

Let us create an example of such a system, using a spreadsheet program and simple data base management and analysis tools, while providing some graphic presentation and trending. This system will relate to the output of the social work department.

One of the more difficult types of productivity to measure is that of the social work department. The measure of the human value of this service is more realistically considered in broader community or societal terms than can be addressed in a book about microcomputer applications. In a larger sense, the value of social work services must be perceived in qualitative terms more than in quantitative terms. However, a simple method of measuring and comparing the quantitative outputs of a social work service, and of doing so with microcomputer assistance, does suggest itself. The quantitative measure of performance is, after all, an important component of any performance measurement system. The application of this method in specific hospital environments must be left to those who have the expertise to do so.

The quantitative method proposed may be used to characterize and monitor the relative outputs or productivity of individual social workers as well as the aggregate output of an entire department. The system permits the development of standards through the collection and analysis of information over a period of time. The standards thus become historically derived within an institution and may be thought of as being dynamic in relation to the dynamic fluctuation of patient mix and patient load. Other environmental factors might also apply to any given hospital's social work milieu.

Case-specific measurement of time spent is the backbone of a social work service productivity measurement system. The tasks required for specific types of cases, or in the performance of activities such as group counseling, can be studied using information produced by a microcomputer-supported system. Procedures for counting individual cases along with their specific characteristics must be established. The forms, procedures, and output reports of any performance measurement system should be established in a way that satisfies the institution's decision-making requirements rather than some information specialist's urge to create a hierarchical structure of conformity for its own sake. This is particularly true for something as difficult to measure as social work activities. The output of the system should be such that it creates comparative information over some period of time. What we want to measure is the mean or median time (or both) required to perform certain types of work or categories of service.

In the sample spreadsheet shown in Exhibit 4-15 the quantitative output of several social workers is analyzed. This report compares the numbers of patients per "degree of difficulty" class arrayed across five such acuity levels for each social worker. Along with this is shown the average age of patients in each class, hours worked by each social worker in dealing with the patient load in each class, hours per patient served, and percent contribution of each class of patient to the worker's total patient load. Forty-two separate calculations are required to produce this report. If information about more social workers were needed, the number of calculations required would increase by 14 per social worker. Creating a report of this type for a staff of ten social workers would require 140 calculations, as well as a large amount of checking, verifying, and correcting. The value of the electronic spreadsheet is clearly indicated in a system when the number of calculations is high or when there is a routine need for the information.

Exhibit 4-15 Productivity Measurement: Social Worker Output

SOCIAL WORK
PRODUCTIVITY REPORT

WORKER BJA

MONTH JAN

PATIENT CLASS	NO PATS	AVG AGE	HRS	HRS/PAT	% CONTR.
CLASS I	28	54	54	1.93	30.11
CLASS II	35	61	77	2.20	37.63
CLASS III	15	64	24	1.60	16.13
CLASS IV	11	71	11	1.00	11.83
CLASS V	4	77	2	0.50	4.30
TOTALS	93		168	1.81	100

SOCIAL WORK
PRODUCTIVITY REPORT

WORKER DAD

MONTH JAN

PATIENT CLASS	NO PATS	AVG AGE	HRS	HRS/PAT	% CONTR.
CLASS I	12	49	16	1.33	15.38
CLASS II	12	57	20	1.67	15.38
CLASS III	14	67	27	1.93	17.95
CLASS IV	32	70	00	2.50	41.03
CLASS V	8	81	25	3.13	10.26
TOTALS	78		168	2.15	100

SOCIAL WORK
PRODUCTIVITY REPORT

WORKER FAG

MONTH JAN

PATIENT CLASS	NO PATS	AVG AGE	HRS	HRS/PAT	% CONTR.
CLASS I	12		24	2.00	15.79
CLASS II	25		45	1.80	32.89
CLASS III	35		82	2.34	46.05
CLASS IV	1		4	4.00	1.32
CLASS V	3		13	4.33	3.95
TOTAL	76		168	2.21	100

An added element of sophistication rests with the department's need to aggregate information on all social workers into a report that directly compares their relative work outputs and effort. The electronic spreadsheet permits the moving of information automatically from one point or "cell" to another. In our example, the totals for each individual social worker are moved by the computer to new locations where additional calculations are made. This new "model" yields a new report containing information that is arrayed in a different way (see Exhibit 4-16).

In addition, comparisons may be made of the relative contributions toward total work effort created by the several patient classes (see Exhibit 4-17) and comparisons of work effort and contribution by worker per patient class. Either of these comparisons can be related to some period or periods of time.

All of this information can be graphed in the manner presented in Figures 4-2, 4-3, and 4-4. The information can be accumulated in a data base over various time periods.

Another dimension may be added to this reporting system by analyzing the totals and averages for the various patient classes and then comparing the information for each worker with these data. More important, the aggregate and individual worker information can be measured over time to determine trends.

These reports, and others of more specific nature, are developed by using a data base that is compiled and stored on disks using the spreadsheet system. Information of the following types may be collected on a monthly basis and aggregated yearly:

- patient intake (number of new cases)
- cases carried over from previous period
- total caseload
- total service hours (including direct service and indirect service)

Exhibit 4-16 Productivity Measurement: Output Comparison

SOCIAL WORK
PRODUCTIVITY REPORT

JAN

WORKER	PATIENTS	AVG AGE	HOURS	HRS/PAT	% TOTAL
BJA	93		168	1.81	37.65
DAD	78		168	2.15	31.58
FAG	76		168	2.21	30.77
TOTAL	247		504	2.04	100.00

Exhibit 4-17 Productivity Measurement: Output by Patient Class

SOCIAL WORK DEPT
PERCENT CONTRIBUTION BY
PATIENT CLASS TO TOTAL WORK EFFORT

MONTH: JAN '83

PATIENT CLASS	NO. PATS	HOURS	HRS/PAT	% PATS CONTR.	% HOURS CONTR.
CLASS I	52	94	1.81	21.05	18.65
CLASS II	72	142	1.97	29.15	28.17
CLASS III	64	133	2.08	25.91	26.39
CLASS IV	44	95	2.16	17.81	18.85
CLASS V	15	40	2.67	6.07	7.94
TOTALS	247	504	2.04	100.00	100.00

Figure 4-2 Social Worker Productivity Measurement: Bar Graph

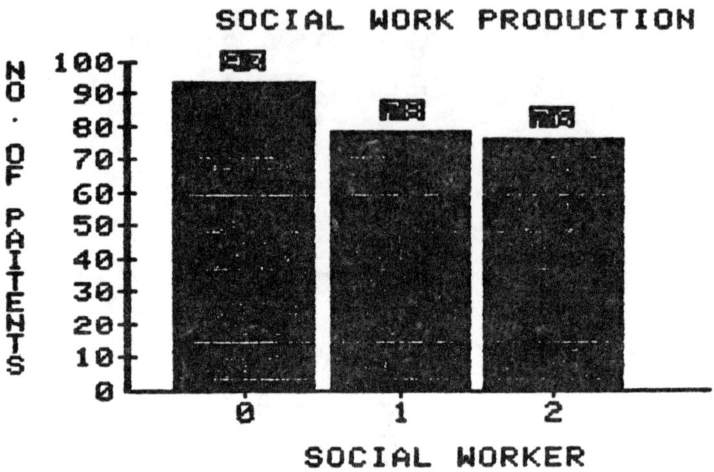

Figure 4-3 Productivity Measurement: Output Comparison Bar Graph

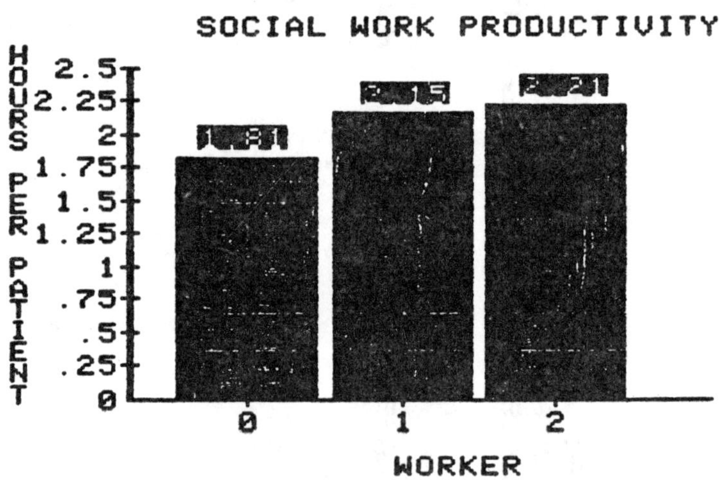

These data may be broken down by number of hours per type of direct patient service such as:

- evaluation
- conference

Figure 4-4 Productivity Measurement: Pie Chart

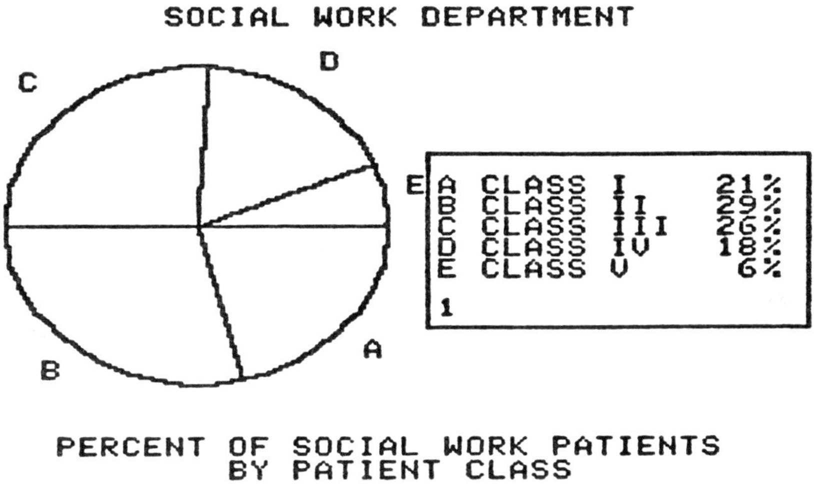

- family service
- consultation
- discharge planning
- community agency planning
- patient/family education

Indirect service can be analyzed by collecting and massaging data on:

- group work (including number of people, number of groups, preparation time, number of sessions, and total sessions)
- sick and vacation period coverage

Other activities, such as department or hospitalwide commitments, research, and community activities can also be factored into the data base, with the number of hours per activity collected for each social worker on a monthly basis. The number of manual calculations avoided using an electronic spreadsheet system could be enormous. The source of all of these data is usually a case card or other data collection form. These data collection documents would be aggregated by a clerk and entered into the spreadsheet format for report production. Exhibit 4-18 shows how the details of the system and the resulting data base would be developed. The

Exhibit 4-18 Productivity Measurement: Data Base

SOCIAL WORK
DATABASE FOR SERVICE CLASSES
DIRECT SERVICE HOURS

1983	J	F	M	A	M	J	J	A	S	O	N	D	T
BJA													
NEW PTS	67	63	64	75	71								341
CARRYOV	22	21	21	25	23								112
SHARED	14	13	13	16	15								71
CLOSED	10	9	10	11	11								51
EVALUAT	23	22	22	26	24								117
CONSULT	12	11	12	13	13								61
CASE CO	8	8	8	9	9								41
FAMILY	14	13	13	16	15								71
PT/FAM	12	11	12	13	13								61
AGENCY	32	30	31	36	34								163
DISCH P	14	13	13	16	15								71
DAD													
NEW PTS	68	64	66	77	73								347
CARRYOV	22	21	22	25	24								114
SHARED	14	13	14	16	15								73
CLOSED	10	10	10	11	11								52
EVALUAT	23	22	22	26	25								119
CONSULT	12	12	12	14	13								62
CASE CO	8	8	8	9	9								41
FAMILY	14	13	14	16	15								73
PT/FAM	12	12	12	14	13								62
AGENCY	33	31	31	37	35								166
DISCH P	14	13	14	16	15								73

FAG													
NEW PTS	65	61	62	73	69								330
CARRYOV	21	20	20	24	23								108
SHARED	14	13	13	15	14								69
CLOSED	10	9	9	11	10								49
EVALUAT	22	21	21	25	24								113
CONSULT	12	11	11	13	12								59
CASE CO	8	7	7	9	8								39
FAMILY	14	13	13	15	14								69
PT/FAM	12	11	11	13	12								59
AGENCY	31	29	30	35	33								158
DISCH P	14	13	13	15	14								69
TOTAL	681	641	653	763	725	0	0	0	0	0	0	0	3464

information contained in the data base can be massaged in many ways to produce reports for analysis by both the department head and administrator.

SPREADSHEET MODELS FOR THE DIETETICS DEPARTMENT

The use of spreadsheets by dietetics department managers and supervisors may be valuable even if the department is not interested in using a more sophisticated system. Consider the following example: the cafeteria manager is interested in knowing the popularity of certain food items offered in the cafeteria line and the amount of waste involved in preparation and serving. It is assumed that the manager has some means of verifying the number of portions served. Many cafeterias now use cash registers that indicate cost based on defined keys; that is, instead of entering $.57 for a serving of corn, the cashier just presses the key marked "corn" and it enters $.57 to the bill.

The first step is to define the items to be tracked; presumably, the more expensive items should be examined first. Then, it is necessary to calculate the number of servings of a particular item to be prepared from a given quantity of basic ingredients.

The spreadsheet is then set up. It may be useful to divide the sheet into different sections corresponding to different sections of the menu. This will allow the calculation of the total number of entrees, the total number of desserts, etc., as well as the percent of the total represented by each item.

At the end of the day, data would be entered into the spreadsheet for all of the food items to be tracked (see Exhibit 4-19).

The spreadsheet shown in Exhibit 4-20 takes these basic numbers and calculates waste costs and loss percentages and amounts. In this case, two reports are prepared separately from one large spreadsheet.

This information could be used, for example, in decision making about which items to offer more or less frequently on the menu or as a means of identifying the need to control costs by revising recipes. It would be a simple matter to graph (for example) the popularity of individual entrees at a meal; this graph is shown in Figure 4-5.

LABOR NEGOTIATIONS INFORMATION SPREADSHEET

One area of personnel management that may be uniquely suited to microcomputer support is that of preparing for and carrying out labor contract negotiations. Of course, personnel involved should be familiar

Exhibit 4-19 Expense Measurement: Food Costs

GENERAL MEMORIAL HOSPITAL
DIETETICS DEPARTMENT
CAFETERIA
SERVINGS PRODUCED VS SERVINGS SOLD

DATE: MAY 31,83

	SERVINGS PRODUCED	SERVINGS SOLD	SERVINGS SAVED	SERVINGS WASTED	COST/ SERVING	WASTE COST	PRICE/ SERVING
ENTREES							
HAM LOAF	230	210	20	0	.94	0.00	1.25
EGGS BENE	120	120	0	0	.82	0.00	1.25
LIVR/ONIO	50	47	0	3	.89	2.67	1.09
SIDES							
POTATOES	300	243	0	57	.35	19.95	0.60
CORN	180	180	0	0	.26	0.00	0.40
WAX BEANS	90	90	0	0	.24	0.00	0.40
CAULIF	50	44	0	6	.35	2.10	0.45
SALAD	125	120	0	5	.23	1.15	0.40
DESSERTS							
APPLE PIE	50	41	9	0	.48	0.00	0.60
PEACH COB	50	32	8	10	.36	3.60	0.50
CH JELLO	80	60	20	0	.18	0.00	0.30
ICE CREAM	30	30	0	0	.25	0.00	0.45
TOTAL	1355	1217	57	81		29.47	

with collective bargaining and its historical impact on institutions. Once the concern of only business and industry, unions are now operating in the public sector and in new arenas such as hospitals. Whereas unions were once mostly made up of craftsmen and other blue-collar laborers, now professionals and technical people are also represented through associations and management must gain expertise in what are often complicated and prolonged labor negotiations. This section will describe ways in which the microcomputer can support management throughout the process of planning for and negotiating a contract.

Exhibit 4-20 Expense Measurement: Sales Analysis

GENERAL MEMORIAL HOSPITAL
DIETETICS DEPARTMENT
CAFETERIA
SALES ANALYSIS

DATE: MAY 31, 1983

	WASTE COST	PERCENT WASTE	PERCENT SOLD	PCT OF GROUP	PROFIT/ (LOSS)
ENTREES					
HAM LOAF	0.00	8.70	91.30	55.70	65.10
EGGS BENE	0.00	0.00	100.00	31.83	51.60
LIVER/ON	2.67	0.00	94.00	12.47	6.73
SIDES					
POTATOES	19.95	0.00	81.00	35.89	40.80
CORN	0.00	0.00	100.00	26.59	25.20
WAX BEANS	0.00	0.00	100.00	13.29	14.40
CAULIF	2.10	0.00	88.00	6.50	2.30
SALAD	1.15	0.00	96.00	17.73	19.25
DESSERTS					
APPLE PIE	0.00	18.00	82.00	25.15	4.92
PEACH COB	3.60	16.00	64.00	19.63	0.88
CH JELLO	0.00	25.00	75.00	36.81	7.20
ICE CREAM	0.00	0.00	100.00	18.40	6.00
	29.47	4.21	89.82		244.38

Contract negotiations determine the wages, hours, and working conditions of the workforce or one of its segments. The result of the negotiations, a statement of the wage and hours bargain and other elements related to workers and management rights and responsibilities, is very important to the ultimate success of a hospital in meeting its service and financial goals.

Our focus is on the ability of management to quickly calculate and project the economic costs of wage and benefit settlements, as well as the costs of other contract provisions. The microcomputer can be put to use in collecting and storing relevant information, often much in advance of the actual negotiations. This can work to great advantage in reaching an agreement that is beneficial to management or in avoiding a potentially costly strike.

During the actual negotiating sessions, which consist of both sides formulating and advancing proposals and counterproposals and (usually) reaching an agreement, management must rely on the best information it

Figure 4-5 Cafeteria Sales: Pie Chart

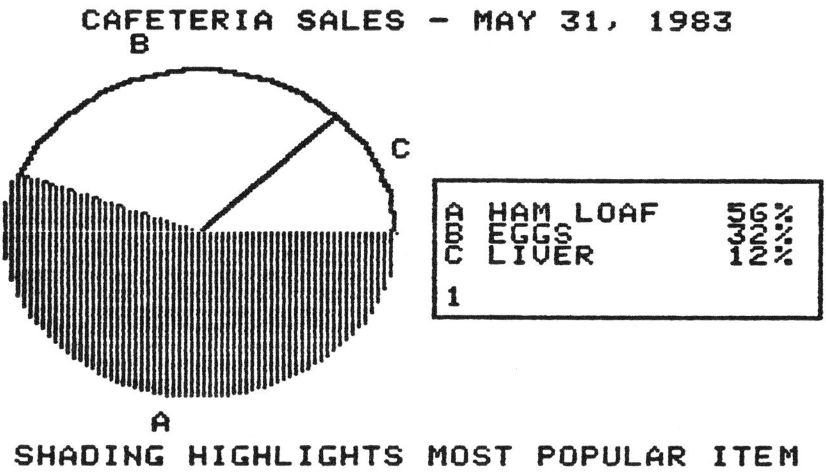

---

can gather. A crucial element is the consideration and acceptance of "last-minute" concessions in order to avoid or end a strike. Such concessions are usually made with little opportunity to analyze or fully understand their future consequences. The rituals of contract negotiations have frequently forced management to live with severe constraints.

It takes many hours to prepare for each actual hour of a contract negotiation session. The information needed both before and during the actual negotiations could well be stored in a microcomputer data base. This can be done either by building a data base from scratch on a micro, which might be the choice of the smaller hospital, or linking the micro to a mainframe-based personnel computer system for purposes of accessing some of the required information. Since most negotiations require extensive fact finding, the resulting information base is likely to be quite large. It could conceivably contain information about:

- current number of employees in the bargaining unit and/or its subdivisions
- current hourly rates
- current benefits and their hourly costs
- current file of statements made by union leaders on issues of relevance
- external factors influencing a union's decisions

- trends in other contracts within the organization
- current grievances
- benchmark information on contracts at other hospitals

Using this information, management can simulate proposals and counterproposals rapidly and with greater confidence in their precision. Cost and other impacts of proposals are more easy to analyze in this manner, and the staff performing the analysis can avoid a certain amount of fatigue. During a marathon negotiating session, the participants often resort to maneuvering intended to affect the agreement outcome to the benefit of their cause. Because bargaining usually takes a competitive form characterized by conflict rather than cooperation, it is necessary to read the real intentions of one's adversary. Failure to do so can result in severe consequences including a strike or agreement to a difficult contract provision. Gauging the purpose of the other side is accomplished more readily when you have timely information. The example below shows how a simple system can be devised to produce some of the required information quickly and accurately both before and during contract negotiations.

The spreadsheet shown in Exhibit 4-21 indicates the types and number of calculations that are capable of being performed in a rapid and accurate manner. Note the ease with which a simple change in the percent of wage increase column can be used to calculate its effect on the potential bottom line financial commitment.

LABOR MARKET ANALYSIS SPREADSHEET

Another use of the microcomputer in the personnel department would be in performing labor market analyses. These analyses are needed to compare salaries currently being paid with those of other institutions. The provision of information by the personnel department to the hospital administration usually requires many hours of preparation. Because this information is most often compiled manually, it must be recalculated each time it is produced. Preparing tables is cumbersome, and one does not often get to see graphic presentations showing trends or tables comparing a number of hospitals because of the time required to prepare them.

Easily devised programs can provide the following information about a hospital's labor force or one of its segments:

- name (and number) of each job classification
- number of employees in each classification

Exhibit 4-21 Financial Simulation: Labor Negotiation

GENERAL MEMORIAL HOSPITAL
PERSONNEL DEPARTMENT RUN DATE: MAY 23,1983

LABOR NEGOTIATION FINANCIAL SIMULATION

JOB TITLE	NUMBER EMPLOYED	HOURLY RATE	ANNUAL HOURS	ANNUAL WAGES	PERCENT FRINGE	TOT WAGES + FRINGE	PERCENT INCREASE	NEW RATE	NEW WAGE+FRIN
BAKER I	9.00	5.86	18360.00	107589.60	0.16	124803.94	.055	6.18	131668
BAKER II	6.00	6.67	12240.00	81640.8	0.16	94703.33	.055	7.04	87779
COOK I	12.00	5.57	24480.00	136353.60	0.16	158170.18	.055	5.88	175558
COOK II	9.00	6.01	18360.00	110343.60	0.16	127998.58	.055	6.34	131668
COOK III	5.00	6.58	10200.00	67116.00	0.16	77854.56	.055	6.94	73149
CUSTODIAN I	32.00	5.34	65280.00	348595.20	0.16	404370.43	.055	5.63	468153
CUSTODIAN II	27.00	5.78	55080.00	318362.40	0.16	369300.38	.055	6.10	395004
CUSTODIAN III	17.00	6.14	34680.00	212935.20	0.16	247004.83	.055	6.48	248707
FOOD SERVICE I	34.00	5.34	69360.00	370382.40	0.16	429643.58	.055	5.63	497413
FOOD SERVICE II	54.00	5.78	110160.00	636724.80	0.16	738600.77	.055	6.10	790009
FOOD SERVICE III	21.00	6.14	42840.00	263037.60	0.16	305123.62	.055	6.48	307226
LAB TECH I	32.00	6.32	65280.00	412569.60	0.16	478580.74	.055	6.67	468153
LAB TECH I	28.00	6.93	57120.00	395841.60	0.16	459176.26	.055	7.31	409634
PATIENT ESCORT	6.00	6.01	12240.00	73562.40	0.16	85332.38	.055	6.34	87779
PHLEBOTOMIST	12.00	7.11	24480.00	174052.80	0.16	201901.25	.055	7.50	175558

Exhibit 4-21 continued

JOB TITLE	NUMBER EMPLOYED	HOURLY RATE	ANNUAL HOURS	ANNUAL WAGES	PERCENT FRINGE	TOT WAGES + FRINGE	PERCENT INCREASE	NEW RATE	NEW WAGE+FRIN
SECURITY GUARD	24.00	6.01	48960.00	294249.60	0.16	341329.54	.055	6.34	351115
STOCKKEEPER I	14.00	5.34	28560.00	152510.40	0.16	176912.06	.055	5.63	204817
STOCKKEEPER II	12.00	5.78	24480.00	141494.40	0.16	164133.50	.055	6.10	175558
WALL WASHER	4.00	6.14	8160.00	50102.40	0.16	58118.78	.055	6.48	58519
BOILERMAKER	1.00	14.88	2040.00	30355.20	0.16	35212.03	.053	15.67	14630
CARPENTER I	6.00	9.55	12240.00	116892.00	0.16	135594.72	.053	10.06	87779
CARPENTER II	4.00	13.65	8160.00	111384.00	0.16	129205.44	.053	14.37	58519
ELECTRICIAN I	7.00	9.55	14280.00	136374.00	0.16	158193.84	.053	10.06	102409
ELECTRICIAN II	7.00	13.65	14280.00	194922.00	0.16	226109.52	.053	14.37	102409
MAINTENANCE	19.00	9.88	38760.00	382948.80	0.16	444220.61	.053	10.40	277966
PLUMBER	3.00	14.43	6120.00	88311.60	0.16	102441.46	.053	15.19	43889
PLUMBER, APPRENTICE	1.00	9.55	2040.00	19482.00	0.16	22599.12	.053	10.06	14630
TOTALS	406.00		828240.00	5428134.00	0.16	6296635.44			5939697

- salary ranges (minimums and maximums for each classification)
- average current salaries for each classification
- average longevity of employees in each classification
- other information as required

Similar information collected in more aggregate terms from other institutions could be entered and compared automatically either using inhouse programming or a program such as the electronic spreadsheet.

Using the mainframe computer for an analysis of this nature would, reasonably, be considered a low priority. It is for this reason that doing this kind of job on a micro is recommended. Downloading the necessary information from a mainframe would require a modest amount of programming but once accomplished this could be used many times. The electronic spreadsheet would take the appearance such as that shown in Exhibit 4-22. The amount of data presented has been limited to keep the example simple. A working system would no doubt contain vastly more data.

SPREADSHEETS TO DETERMINE STAFFING NEEDS

Another area in which microcomputers can be of significant use in managing the housekeeping services for a hospital is that of projecting appropriate staff levels for a defined area.

This can be accomplished by first defining a set of rooms for inspection and cost projection that will fit into the computer program to be used. Let us make use of the spreadsheet program to create a simulation model of the services to be offered in each space.

Each of the rooms should be examined with regard to the services to be performed. Several categories will emerge based on the services offered. In the example shown in Exhibit 4-23 the number of categories has been limited to only three: Patient Room, Utility, and Office. Spreadsheet programs are capable of handling a full range of categories.

The next step is to completely define all of the tasks to be performed in the categories set aside; these tasks should be defined in terms of both the basic time unit for the service and the number of units required to perform the service in a given space. For example, if the custodian needs to sweep the floor in a space every day and it takes him 10 minutes to sweep 200 square feet, the appropriate numbers required for a room with 250 square feet of floor area are as follows: time unit, .16 hours; units required, 2.5.

It is a good idea to make a standard time unit and a standard unit of space for all categories; for example, you may want to provide standards based on every 100 square feet of area and cost based on hours of effort.

Exhibit 4-22 Labor Market Analysis: Allied Health Classes

GENERAL MEMORIAL HOSPITAL
PERSONNEL DEPARTMENT
LABOR MARKET ANALYSIS

ALLIED HEALTH CLASS

JOB TITLE	SAL CLASS	SALARY RANGE		NUMBER OF EMPLOYEES	AVG CURR SALARY	AVG YRS SERVICE	CURRENT AVERAGE SALARY REGION1	REGION 2	REGION 3
CARDIOPULM TECH	AH-09	15600	19600	9	17600	4	18128	18832	18480
DIETITIAN I	AH-06	12300	14900	3	13600	2	14008	14552	14280
DIETITIAN II	AH-08	14800	17200	8	16000	4	16480	17120	16800
DIETITIAN III	AH-10	17200	21900	4	19550	7	20137	20919	20528
EEG TECH	AH-09	15600	19600	3	17600	4	18128	18832	18480
EKG TECH	AH-09	15600	19600	4	17600	3	18128	18832	18480
HEALTH REC ANALYST	AH-07	13700	16400	12	15050	5	15502	16104	15803
NUCLEAR MED TECH	AH-08	14800	17200	3	16000	5	16480	17120	16800
PHARMACY TECH	AH-05	11700	14300	4	13000	6	13390	13910	13650
RADIOLOGY TECHNICIAN	AH-08	14800	17200	7	16000	5	16480	17120	16800
RADIOL TECHNOLOGIST	AH-10	17200	21900	5	19550	2	20137	20919	20528
RESP THERAPY TECH	AH-05	11700	14300	8	13000	4	13390	13910	13650
RESP THERAPIST	AH-09	15600	19600	3	17600	4	18128	18832	18480
SOCIAL WORKER I	AH-08	14800	17200	3	16000	2	16480	17120	16800
SOCIAL WORKER II	AH-10	17200	21900	2	19550	5	20137	20919	20528

Exhibit 4-23 Projecting Staffing Needs: Housekeeping

PRODUCT MEASURES
BASED ON RATIOS OF
ACTUAL TO STANDARD
HOURS

HOUSEKEEPING
MAY, 1983

MEASURES	QUANTITY	STANDARD HOURS	ACTUAL HOURS	% PROD. STD=100
TOT. ROOMS CLEANED	2205			
STANDARD ROOMS	1145			
CUSTOM ROOMS	701			
DELUXE ROOMS	359			
BASIC HRS/RM STD	.5	1102.5	1068	103.23
CUSTOM HRS/RM STD	.1	70.1	95	73.79
DELUXE HRS/RM STD	.2	71.8	85	84.47
TOT. HRS		1244.4	1248	99.71
RATIOS				
AV CLEANING HRS/RM		0.56	0.57	99.71
ROOMS CLEANED/HR		1.77	1.77	100

There are, of course, services provided that are not based on square feet, for example, window blind cleaning. In this area, we will approximate this service. However, it would be possible to develop a sufficiently detailed model that would provide an even more accurate projection; it would then be necessary to go to all spaces involved and count windows, sinks, ashtrays, etc.

It is not our intention to provide a complete guide to the subject of preparing a time study with regard to housekeeping; there are standard texts available. Also, prepared standards are available through such organizations as the Executive Housekeepers Association; you may wish to check the *Encyclopedia of Associations* in the library.

At this point, the user must distinguish between the cost of each time unit of effort. Hospitals with unionized labor forces typically have different job classifications at different pay rates. Each job class has a defined set of duties. The tasks required in a room may call for labor of two or more pay classifications but this can easily be factored into the growing simulation model. Exhibit 4-24 illustrates the steps taken thus far.

The cost of the labor required, in the form of a per hour (or per unit, if a different time unit has been defined) should be placed in the column following time per task.

Exhibit 4-24 Projecting Staffing Needs: Labor Requirements Template

HOUSEKEEPING DEPARTMENT
LABOR REQUIREMENTS SUMMARY

	UNIT	ROOM 2301	ROOM 2303	ROOM 2305
LABOR #1				
CLEAN BED	HOUR	0.00	0.00	0.00
CHANGE BED		0.00	0.00	0.00
CLN COUNTR		0.00	0.00	0.00
CLN BATHR		0.00	0.00	0.00
TOTAL		0.00	0.00	0.00
LABOR #2				
CLEAN FLR		0.00	0.00	0.00
MOP FLR		0.00	0.00	0.00
PULL TRASH		0.00	0.00	0.00
TOTAL		0.00	0.00	0.00
LABOR #3				
WASH WALLS		0.00	0.00	0.00
WASH WINDW		0.00	0.00	0.00
TOTAL		0.00	0.00	0.00
LABOR #4				
DISCHARGE		0.00	0.00	0.00
HI DUST		0.00	0.00	0.00
TOTAL		0.00	0.00	0.00

Next the room numbers of the spaces considered in this projection effort are added. Finally, using the physical characters of the space in conjunction with the standards established for each task, the number of time units required is filled in in the appropriate space under each room. The result is shown in Exhibit 4-25.

Obviously, this table has only a limited value by itself. It is easy, however, with VisiCalc, to build an additional table on the same spreadsheet to provide useful summary information with respect to the tasks and hours required. The table shown in Exhibit 4-26 uses the information to yield a per room cost for housekeeping service.

The same technique can be used to summarize the staffing needs for the defined rooms by simply multiplying the number of hours required per cleaning times the number of days to be cleaned in the year to provide an annual full time equivalent for any space. This table is shown in Exhibit 4-27, which is just below the table in Exhibit 4-26 on the VisiCalc sheet.

Exhibit 4-25 Projecting Staffing Needs: Labor Requirements Summary

HOUSEKEEPING DEPARTMENT
LABOR REQUIREMENTS SUMMARY

	UNIT	ROOM 2301	ROOM 2303	ROOM 2305
LABOR #1				
CLEAN BED	HOUR	0.10	0.10	0.00
CHANGE BED		0.14	0.14	0.00
CLN COUNTR		0.06	0.10	0.05
CLN BATHR		0.19	0.22	0.20
TOTAL		0.49	0.56	0.25
LABOR #2				
CLEAN FLR		0.12	0.14	0.13
MOP FLR		0.10	0.11	0.12
PULL TRASH		0.02	0.02	0.02
TOTAL		0.24	0.27	0.27
LABOR #3				
WASH WALLS		0.08	0.07	0.09
WASH WINDW		0.02	0.04	0.04
TOTAL		0.10	0.11	0.13
LABOR #4				
DISCHARGE		0.24	0.24	0.00
HI DUST		0.05	0.07	0.07
TOTAL		0.29	0.31	0.07

There is an additional benefit of having this information on an electronic, rather than paper, spreadsheet. Suppose a salesman came to your department and offered to sell you a device that could allow your department to clean floors more efficiently. Given a time savings figure, you could easily fold it into the information contained in the first table, and the rest of the dependent formulas in the other tables would be calculated automatically, providing an accurate, detailed assessment of the value of the new technique or product.

This same method can be applied to the housekeeping supplies to be used on a unit in the course of a year. By defining the supplies to be used on a unit (or in a room) an appropriate projection could be made. Exhibit 4-28 illustrates this kind of approach with a unit level summary for a portion of a hospital. The totals at the end of the row indicate the total volume and cost of each supply. This sort of summary makes purchasing decisions regarding materials much easier, particularly with regard to volume-based discounts.

Exhibit 4-26 Cost Projection: Housekeeping Parts and Labor per Room

HOUSEKEEPING DEPARTMENT
INDIVIDUAL ROOM CLEANING COST PROJECTION

PARTS AND LABOR	UNIT COST	ROOM 2301 # UNITS	COST	ROOM 2303 # UNITS	COST	ROOM 2305 # UNITS	COST
PAPER TOWL	0.35	0.75	0.26	0.70	0.25	0.65	0.23
SOAP TISSU	2.54	0.10	0.25	0.20	0.51	0.50	1.27
TOILET PPR	0.23	0.50	0.12	0.10	0.02	0.00	0.00
TISSUES	0.21	0.25	0.05	0.00	0.00	0.75	0.16
TRASH BAG	0.01	2.00	0.02	2.00	0.02	3.00	0.03
CLNG SPRAY	1.45	0.25	0.36	0.25	0.36	0.35	0.51
LABOR #1	5.05	0.49	2.47	0.56	2.83	0.25	1.26
LABOR #2	5.45	0.24	1.31	0.27	1.47	0.27	1.47
LABOR #3	5.95	0.10	0.60	0.11	0.65	0.13	0.77
LABOR #4	6.45	0.29	1.87	0.31	2.00	0.07	0.45
TOTAL COST PER ROOM PER CLEANING			7.31		8.11		6.15

SUMMARY OF ROOM CLEANINGS
FOR ONE YEAR

	ONE	TWO	THREE	WEEKLY CLEANING
TIMES CLEANED/WEEK	7.00	7.00	5.00	1.00

MONTH	WEEKS CLEANED	RM 2301 COSTS	TIMES CLEANED	RM 2303 COSTS	TIMES CLEANED	RM 2301 COSTS	TIMES CLEANED	TOTAL COST
COST PER WEEK		51.20	56.78	30.76	138.74			
JANUARY	4.00	204.81	28.00	227.14	28.00	123.03	20.00	554.97
FEBRUARY	4.00	204.81	28.00	227.14	28.00	123.03	20.00	554.97
MARCH	5.00	256.01	35.00	283.92	35.00	153.79	25.00	693.72
APRIL	4.00	204.81	28.00	227.14	28.00	123.03	20.00	554.97
MAY	4.00	204.81	28.00	227.14	28.00	123.03	20.00	554.97
JUNE	5.00	256.01	35.00	283.92	35.00	153.79	25.00	693.72
JULY	4.00	204.81	28.00	227.14	28.00	123.03	20.00	554.97
AUGUST	5.00	256.01	35.00	283.92	35.00	153.79	25.00	693.72
SEPTEMBER	4.00	204.81	28.00	227.14	28.00	123.03	20.00	554.97
OCTOBER	4.00	204.81	28.00	227.14	28.00	123.03	20.00	554.97
NOVEMBER	5.00	256.01	35.00	283.92	35.00	153.79	25.00	693.72
DECEMBER	4.00	204.81	28.00	227.14	28.00	123.03	20.00	554.97
	52.00	2662.48	364.00	2952.77	364.00	1599.39	260.00	7214.64

Exhibit 4-27 Projecting Staffing Needs: Labor Requirements Summary

ANNUAL LABOR
REQUIREMENTS

	LABOR #1	LABOR #2	LABOR #3	LABOR #4
JANUARY	34.40	19.68	8.48	18.20
FEBRUARY	34.40	19.68	8.48	18.20
MARCH	43.00	24.60	10.60	22.75
APRIL	34.40	19.68	8.48	18.20
MAY	34.40	19.68	8.48	18.20
JUNE	43.00	24.60	10.60	22.75
JULY	34.40	19.68	8.48	18.20
AUGUST	43.00	24.60	10.60	22.75
SEPTEMBER	34.40	19.68	8.48	18.20
OCTOBER	34.40	19.68	8.48	18.20
NOVEMBER	43.00	24.60	10.60	22.75
DECEMBER	34.40	19.68	8.48	18.20
TOTALS	447.20	255.84	110.24	236.60

* ALL FIGURES IN HOURS

Exhibit 4-28 Projecting Costs: Materials Requirements

ANNUAL MATERIALS
REQUIREMENTS

	PAPER TWL	SOAP TIS	TOILET P	TISSUES	TRASH BG	CLNG SPR
JANUARY	53.60	18.40	16.80	22.00	172.00	21.00
FEBRUARY	53.60	18.40	16.80	22.00	172.00	21.00
MARCH	67.00	23.00	21.00	27.50	215.00	26.25
APRIL	53.60	18.40	16.80	22.00	172.00	21.00
MAY	53.60	18.40	16.80	22.00	172.00	21.00
JUNE	67.00	23.00	21.00	27.50	215.00	26.25
JULY	53.60	18.40	16.80	22.00	172.00	21.00
AUGUST	67.00	23.00	21.00	27.50	215.00	26.25
SEPTEMBER	53.60	18.40	16.80	22.00	172.00	21.00
OCTOBER	53.60	18.40	16.80	22.00	172.00	21.00
NOVEMBER	67.00	23.00	21.00	27.50	215.00	26.25
DECEMBER	53.60	18.40	16.80	22.00	172.00	21.00
TOTAL	696.80	239.20	218.40	286.00	2236.00	273.00

SPREADSHEETS FOR BUDGET CONTROL AND FORECASTING

Unit Finances and Activity

We will begin by examining a simple system that will allow easy modeling of the finances and activity of a hospital inpatient unit.

Exhibit 4-29 is a "zeroed" copy of the electronic spreadsheet to be used. This spreadsheet consists of five sections, each of which examines a particular part of the inpatient unit budget. The first section consists of a statement of activity over a fiscal year, expressed (in this example) in patient days. The activity is totaled at the end of the row for the fiscal year.

The second section, STRAIGHT LINE EXPENSES, handles the payroll-related charges incurred by a unit budget. Note that this model can be easily modified to fit the accounting system used in a particular hospital. Each payroll expense is divided into actual salary expense and additional expense in the form of sick and vacation support for the positions involved. The expense for each class is totaled by month and by year.

The third section, PATIENT DAY RELATED EXPENSES, is divided into all expense classes that have been identified as being historically related to patient days in some way. For example, there is a direct correspondence between the number of patient days associated with a given inpatient unit and the cost of medical/surgical supplies for that area. This correspondence is determined by examining past activity to determine the degree and reliability of correspondence. Each expense class is given an index, expressed in dollars per patient day, which is a number expressing the ratio of expense to activity as it has occurred in the past. For example, if the last 10,000 patient days have been accompanied by a $35,000 expense in medical/surgical supplies, the index would be $35,000 divided by 10,000 patient days, or $3.50/patient day. Each expense class is totaled by fiscal year and the section is totaled by month.

There are, of course, many supplies in each budget category that are not related to patient days. Some constitute a fixed expense, while others may more likely be related to admissions (i.e., each patient gets one such item). The formulas for this section could be easily modified to take advantage of the degree of knowledge possessed by the individual user; for example, budgeted admissions could be added under patient days. Patient-day related statistics could be modified to include this additional data.

Historically derived indices are also an adequate forecasting device but it is better to use data related to supply usage. Price indices taken from

Exhibit 4-29 Budget Control: Inpatient Unit

HOSPITAL OPERATIONS
BUDGET PROJECTION FOR FISCAL YEAR:
FOR ACCOUNT NUMBER: 198765
ACCOUNT NAME: TWO WEST OPERATIONS

	JULY	AUG	SEPT	OCT	NOV	DEC	JAN	FEB	MAR	APR	MAY	JUN	TOTAL
BUDGETED PT. DAY	0	0	0	0	0	0	0	0	0	0	0	0	0

STRAIGHT LINE EXPENSES

EXPENSE CLASS	JULY	AUG	SEPT	OCT	NOV	DEC	JAN	FEB	MAR	APR	MAY	JUN	TOTAL
PROF. AND ADMIN.	0	0	0	0	0	0	0	0	0	0	0	0	0
SICK/VAC	0	0	0	0	0	0	0	0	0	0	0	0	0
TOTAL	0	0	0	0	0	0	0	0	0	0	0	0	0
AFSCME	0	0	0	0	0	0	0	0	0	0	0	0	0
SICK/VAC	0	0	0	0	0	0	0	0	0	0	0	0	0
LONGEVITY	0	0	0	0	0	0	0	0	0	0	0	0	0
TOTAL	0	0	0	0	0	0	0	0	0	0	0	0	0
OFFICE	0	0	0	0	0	0	0	0	0	0	0	0	0
SICK/VAC	0	0	0	0	0	0	0	0	0	0	0	0	0
TOTAL	0	0	0	0	0	0	0	0	0	0	0	0	0
OTHER PAY	0	0	0	0	0	0	0	0	0	0	0	0	0
MONTHLY TOTALS	0	0	0	0	0	0	0	0	0	0	0	0	0

PATIENT DAY RELATED EXPENSES

EXPENSE CLASS	INDEX	JULY	AUG	SEPT	OCT	NOV	DEC	JAN	FEB	MAR	APR	MAY	JUN	TOTAL
GEN & OFFICE	1.2356	0	0	0	0	0	0	0	0	0	0	0	0	0
MED/SURG	6.8321	0	0	0	0	0	0	0	0	0	0	0	0	0
PHARMACY	3.1928	0	0	0	0	0	0	0	0	0	0	0	0	0
LIN-BED-LAUNDRY	2.7687	0	0	0	0	0	0	0	0	0	0	0	0	0
MONTHLY TOTALS		0	0	0	0	0	0	0	0	0	0	0	0	0

SPECIAL SCHEDULE EXPENSES

EXPENSE CLASS	JULY	AUG	SEPT	OCT	NOV	DEC	JAN	FEB	MAR	APR	MAY	JUN	TOTAL
CONTRACT SERV.	0	0	0	0	0	0	0	0	0	0	0	0	0
POSTAGE	0	0	0	0	0	0	0	0	0	0	0	0	0
TELEPHONE	0	0	0	0	0	0	0	0	0	0	0	0	0
FOOD	0	0	0	0	0	0	0	0	0	0	0	0	0
MONTHLY TOTALS	0	0	0	0	0	0	0	0	0	0	0	0	0
MONTHLY PAYROLL EXP.	0	0	0	0	0	0	0	0	0	0	0	0	0
MONTHLY COMMODIT EXP.	0	0	0	0	0	0	0	0	0	0	0	0	0
TOTAL MONTHLY EXP.	0	0	0	0	0	0	0	0	0	0	0	0	0

TOTAL PAYROLL EXPENSE	0
TOTAL COMMODITY EXPENSE	0
TOTAL EXPENSE	0

previous years may not be applicable to future years because of the inflationary increase in the cost of medical supplies. A careful examination of the prices of a selection of the items contributing the most to the expenses charged to a unit can provide a more accurate index for that expense class; however, because the cost increases for medical supplies vary widely from one supply to another, this method carries with it an inherent inaccuracy. If a reasonably accurate projection of inflation can be made, simply multiply the derived index times the inflation rate plus 100 percent.

The entries under SPECIAL SCHEDULE EXPENSES are neither straight line nor visibly related to any activity indicator. A good example is found in the expenses associated with contract services; a fee for groundskeeping or plant maintenance may be paid once per year, at the beginning of the fiscal year. A simple straight line budget, with the budgeted funds spread evenly over the year, would show an artificial unfavorable variance because of the large single expenditure.

The final section provides the monthly and annual totals for payroll and commodity for the entire account. This section is created by using a special formula incorporating the subtotals from the earlier sections.

Notice the use of the activity indicators from the top row of the form. The activity figures are placed before the area in which they are to be used because of the order of calculation of the program. If the user does not want information used in preparing a report to appear in the report, the information is simply entered outside the area of the spreadsheet to be printed.

This program can be used for both budget control and for projecting costs on a unit-by-unit basis. The following procedure should be followed when entering and using this report:

1. Boot the spreadsheet program disk; make sure that you have a storage diskette initialized to store the finished sheet.
2. Make sure that the column setting is correct.
3. Begin entering all necessary labels.
4. Enter formulas as indicated in Exhibit 4-29.
5. Save the zeroed spreadsheet on the storage disk.
6. Enter data for a particular fiscal year.
7. Check for the accuracy of the program, particularly the range of formulas.
8. Save the finished sheet on the diskette.

Having entered the data for a unit and fiscal year, be sure to name the spreadsheet; also, a revision date should be added. This sheet can then be saved under a filename different from the zeroed sheet, so it can be called up later.

The spreadsheet along with the activity figures provides a cost projection tool as well as a means of budget control. Begin by printing out a copy of the spreadsheet as it currently exists. Then use your knowledge of the situation to begin projecting the possible outcomes of the year's activity. For example, if you are told to project the budgetary consequences of a construction project that would last from August to November and reduce patient days by 35 percent, have the machine multiply the patient day figures for those months by .65; the end result is automatically added. Additional pieces of data can be factored in using the same sort of method. The user should take care, however, not to disturb any existing formulas.

Once completed, the spreadsheet can be saved to disk to provide a readily accessible data base; it can also be printed to provide the user with hard copy. It is a good idea to type (perhaps at the bottom of the spreadsheet) the assumptions used in creating a particular projection; this statement may or may not be printed out on the spreadsheet.

YTD Charges and Activity

Spreadsheet programs also provide an ideal method for the forecasting of year-end expense based on year-to-date charges and activity. Exhibit 4-30 shows a simple worksheet used to illustrate the variances between actual expense and three different budgets: the first provided by the central accounting department, the second a straight line budget, and the third based on patient days.

Administrative Summaries

Another ideal application for the spreadsheet program is in the area of administrative summaries that must be provided for large-scale new program studies and other budget control efforts. Exhibit 4-31 illustrates a projected budget for a new program to be implemented in a small hospital. The example shows a balance sheet for the major financial areas within the hospital itself, separated into indirect and direct operating expenses; direct operating expenses are those that contribute to revenue.

The individual columns show, for each area, the projected transfer of budgeted funds from areas centralized under the new program, the existing budgets for each department, the incremental increase necessary under the new program, and the associated equipment purchase costs. The bottom portion of the page indicates the final totals for summary presentation.

Exhibit 4-30 Forecasting Expenses: YTD Charges and Activity

GENERAL HOSPITAL
BUDGET VARIANCE REPORT
MONTH OF APRIL, 1983

EXP. CLASS	ACTUAL	ACCTNG BUDGET	DOLLAR	PERCENT	STRT.	DOLLAR	PERCENT	PAT. DAYS	DOLLAR	PERCENT
PRO & ADM	1357.20	1456.23	99.03	6.80	1312.45	-44.75	-3.41	1259.95	-97.25	-7.72
AFSCME	2413.56	2365.70	-47.86	-2.02	2241.55	-172.01	-7.67	2151.89	-261.67	-12.16
OFFICE	890.23	756.76	-133.47	-17.64	892.24	2.01	0.23	856.55	-33.68	-3.93
OTHER PAY	123.54	231.44	107.90	46.62	195.86	72.32	36.92	188.03	64.49	34.30
POSTAGE	23.44	43.56	20.12	46.19	12.50	-10.94	-87.52	12.00	-11.44	-95.33
TEL & TEL	145.88	125.65	-20.23	-16.10	1119.42	973.54	86.97	1074.65	928.77	86.43
FOOD	14.55	54.76	40.21	73.43	9.85	-4.70	-47.72	9.46	-5.09	-53.87
GENERAL	453.77	756.43	302.66	40.01	485.12	31.35	6.46	465.72	11.95	2.56
PHARMACY	1288.98	678.54	-610.44	-89.96	1195.44	-93.54	-7.82	1147.62	-141.36	-12.32
LINEN	1564.65	1243.91	-320.74	-25.78	1595.30	30.65	1.92	1531.49	-33.16	-2.17
MED/SURG	3145.34	2514.65	-630.69	-25.08	3542.18	396.84	11.20	3400.49	255.15	7.50
TOTAL	11421.14	10227.63	-1193.51	-11.67	12601.91	1180.77	9.37	12097.84	676.70	5.59

Exhibit 4-31 Forecasting Expenses: New Programs

Hospital Operations
Financial Summary

Indirect Operating Expenses (Expressed in thousands)	Transfer	Existing	Incrmnt.	Equip.
Plant – (In thousands)				
Maintenance/Alterations	0.00	100.00	14.20	1.20
Housekeeping	0.00	42.50	15.32	2.15
Protective Services	8.00	11.20	3.20	0.00
Equipment Depreciation	0.00	16.30	2.40	0.00
Building Depreciation	0.00	31.55	21.40	0.00
Rent (received)	0.00	0.00	0.00	0.00
Subtotal	8.00	201.55	56.52	3.35
Other – (in thousands)				
Admitting	3.55	21.65	15.84	1.50
Ambulance	4.50	8.12	0.00	21.50
Furnishings	0.00	0.00	0.00	125.10
Hospital Administration	0.00	24.31	0.00	2.10
Unit Management	0.00	43.12	16.13	2.00
Medical Records	0.00	0.00	21.00	1.00
Subtotal	8.05	97.20	52.97	153.20

Exhibit 4-31 continued

Direct Operating Expenses (Expressed in thousands)	Transfer	Existing	Incrmnt.	Equip.
Anesthesiology	0.00	156.43	75.50	86.70
Nursing	35.50	251.50	21.50	12.50
Operating Room	176.30	153.30	189.50	55.40
Radiology	0.00	15.30	15.30	54.60
Social work	0.00	12.50	12.50	3.00
Subtotal	211.80	589.03	314.30	212.20
Expense Total	227.85	887.78	423.79	368.75

In order to provide a simple break-even analysis of this program, a revenue projection summary similar to the expense projection is needed. Exhibit 4-32 shows an analysis of the revenue projected. Figures are presented in fiscal 1982 dollars. The final page of this report is shown in Exhibit 4-33, summarizing the overall revenue and expense picture for the year following the implementation of the program.

A particularly nice feature of spreadsheet programs is that one of the most annoying problems associated with preparing a summary report of this kind is eliminated. Because the individual figures are typically provided by individual departments, each with its own priorities, it is difficult to obtain the final, revised, complete figures. A summary sheet like the one shown may go through many last-minute changes; the program can calculate the new sheet in seconds and print a fresh new copy in less than a minute.

New Program Impact

We will now explore several methods of projecting financial and activity data using the spreadsheet program developed earlier in this chapter. As we have seen, the spreadsheets placed on the computer are more than just static statements of a particular account or area. They can be used as a basis or springboard for exploring the possibilities of the situation.

The spreadsheet shown in Exhibit 4-34 illustrates the situation in a particular inpatient unit account. It is a simple matter to use this sheet to play a "What if . . ." game with this account. For example, what effect would a new program implemented in this unit have on the cost of running the unit? Consider the following new program for our hypothetical unit:

- Program is to start in September, to continue indefinitely.
- Approximately 15 new patients per month are expected, staying about 11 days each.
- Patients would require a more acute form of care.
- Special medical supplies must be given to each patient, costing $25.00 each. These must be changed daily.

Exhibit 4-34 shows the current financial picture for this unit. Let us begin by breaking down the impact that this program will have on unit expenses into the following areas: (1) impact on patient days, (2) impact on personnel, and (3) impact on supplies.

Since we know that there will be about 15 new patients per month staying about 11 days each, approximately 165 patient days will be added

Exhibit 4-32 Revenue Projection: Hospital Operations

Hospital Operations
Financial Summary

Gross Revenue Source (Expressed in thousands)	FY82 (proj)	FY83 (proj)
Patient Unit *	1273.00	1489.00
Operating Rooms	325.00	548.00
Anesthesiology Equipment Fees	25.00	32.00
Radiology	16.50	42.40
Respiratory Therapy	12.00	32.50
Laboratory Tests	35.60	52.90
Total	1687.10	2196.80

* Figure based on projection from the first eight months of activity in the past fiscal year.

Exhibit 4-33 Revenue Projection: Summary Report

```
Hospital Operations
Financial Summary

Expense versus Revenue


                                        FY82 (Proj)          FY83 (Proj)

Gross Revenue                               1687.10              2196.80
(All figures in thousands)
Direct Operating Expense                    1115.63              1429.93
                                           --------             --------
       Operating Contribution                571.47               766.87
Operating Indirect Expense                   314.80               424.29
                                           --------             --------
       Gross Margin                          256.67               342.58
```

Exhibit 4-34 Operating Expenses: Inpatient Unit

HOSPITAL OPERATIONS
BUDGET PROJECTION FOR FISCAL YEAR:
FOR ACCOUNT NUMBER: 198765
ACCOUNT NAME: TWO WEST OPERATIONS

	JULY	AUG	SEPT	OCT	NOV	DEC	JAN	FEB	MAR	APR	MAY	JUN	TOTAL
BUDGETED PT. DAY	678	699	657	701	644	456	477	633	687	675	732	743	7782

STRAIGHT LINE EXPENSES

EXPENSE CLASS	JULY	AUG	SEPT	OCT	NOV	DEC	JAN	FEB	MAR	APR	MAY	JUN	TOTAL
PROF. AND ADMIN.	2155	2155	2155	2155	2155	2155	2155	2155	2155	2155	2155	2155	25860
SICK/VAC	110	110	110	110	110	110	110	110	110	110	110	110	1320
TOTAL	2265	2265	2265	2265	2265	2265	2265	2265	2265	2265	2265	2265	27180
AFSCME	4231	4231	4231	4231	4231	4231	4231	4231	4231	4231	4231	4231	50772
SICK/VAC	215	215	215	215	215	215	215	215	215	215	215	215	2580
LONGEVITY	38	38	38	38	38	38	38	38	38	38	38	38	456
TOTAL	4484	4484	4484	4484	4484	4484	4484	4484	4484	4484	4484	4484	53808
OFFICE	1890	1890	1890	1890	1890	1890	1890	1890	1890	1890	1890	1890	22680
SICK/VAC	85	85	85	85	85	85	85	85	85	85	85	85	1020
TOTAL	1975	1975	1975	1975	1975	1975	1975	1975	1975	1975	1975	1975	23700
OTHER PAY	145	145	145	145	145	145	145	145	145	145	145	145	1740
MONTHLY TOTALS	8869	8869	8869	8869	8869	8869	8869	8869	8869	8869	8869	8869	106428

PATIENT DAY RELATED EXPENSES

EXPENSE CLASS	INDEX	JULY	AUG	SEPT	OCT	NOV	DEC	JAN	FEB	MAR	APR	MAY	JUN	TOTAL
GEN & OFFICE	1.2356	838	864	812	866	796	563	589	782	849	834	904	918	9615
MED/SURG	6.8321	4632	4776	4489	4789	4400	3115	3259	4325	4694	4612	5001	5076	53167
PHARMACY	3.1928	2165	2232	2098	2238	2056	1456	1523	2021	2193	2155	2337	2372	24846
LIN-BED-LAUNDRY	2.7687	1877	1935	1819	1941	1783	1263	1321	1753	1902	1869	2027	2057	21546
MONTHLY TOTALS		9512	9806	9217	9834	9035	6397	6692	8880	9638	9470	10269	10424	109175

SPECIAL SCHEDULE EXPENSES

EXPENSE CLASS	JULY	AUG	SEPT	OCT	NOV	DEC	JAN	FEB	MAR	APR	MAY	JUN	TOTAL
CONTRACT SERV.	256	155	876	456	34	145	321	564	134	55	467	976	4439
POSTAGE	44	34	34	45	23	23	23	44	55	33	44	88	490
TELEPHONE	4533	177	188	165	176	156	176	165	188	156	378	267	6726
FOOD	35	48	47	26	58	36	48	25	18	37	48	154	580
MONTHLY TOTALS	4868	414	1145	693	291	360	568	798	395	281	937	1485	12235
MONTHLY PAYROLL EXP.	8869	8869	8869	8869	8869	8869	8869	8869	8869	8869	8869	8869	106428
MONTHLY COMMODIT EXP.	14380	10220	10362	10527	9326	6757	7260	9678	10033	9751	11206	11909	121410
TOTAL MONTHLY EXP.	23249	19089	19231	19396	18195	15626	16129	18547	18902	18620	20075	20778	227838

TOTAL PAYROLL EXPENSE	106428
TOTAL COMMODITY EXPENSE	121410
TOTAL EXPENSE	227838

to the unit's total expected patient days. Typically, admissions drop in December; let's add only 100 patient days to that month. The changes should be made directly into each cell.

The impact on personnel is more difficult to predict. If this budget includes just nurses and clericals, it becomes a little bit easier, but more information is needed. At this point, you may call the nurse staffing office (or the unit head nurse) and find that an additional two or three patients per day will require an additional nurse on weekends, evenings, and midnights. On this particular unit (let us suppose), the census normally drops considerably on weekends, with patients requiring relatively little care.

No increase in clerical cost is anticipated; additional nursing costs are added under straight line expenses.

Since the patient requires a more acute form of care than that presently provided, the cost per patient-day index will go up for patient-day related expenses. Because we do not know exactly how much (it may not be precisely determinable), we are forced to estimate by using information that may be available for similar patients elsewhere in the hospital, and then combine it for the patient mix expected.

Also, we know that a special medical supply will be required, one that is closely tied to patient days. This cost can be folded into the increased med/surg budget or a special category can be created, showing both the day-by-day cost and the cost of purchasing an initial stock of the items in question. In the example shown, the supply was found to come in boxes of 100 per case.

The result is seen in Exhibit 4-35; it gives a clear picture of the variance to be expected or, alternatively, the funding that must be made available to the unit to balance expenses for the unit. The variance can also be graphed; Figure 4-6 shows the original budget projection and the projection plus new program, graphed against each other. The effect of the new program on the annual expense budget is shown in the graph in Figure 4-7, which plots the cumulative expense for the two budgets.

Using Graphics

The spreadsheets and graphics for this book were both produced on VisiCalc and VisiTrend/Plot, both products of VisiCorp. Because these programs were written to communicate with each other via text files, it was possible to transfer the data from the two spreadsheets directly to the VisiTrend/Plot program. Once in the VisiTrend/Plot program, the cumulative budget figures were prepared using the Trend routines. The two graphs were then prepared and saved to a diskette file pending printing.

Figure 4-6 New Program Impact: Projection Graph

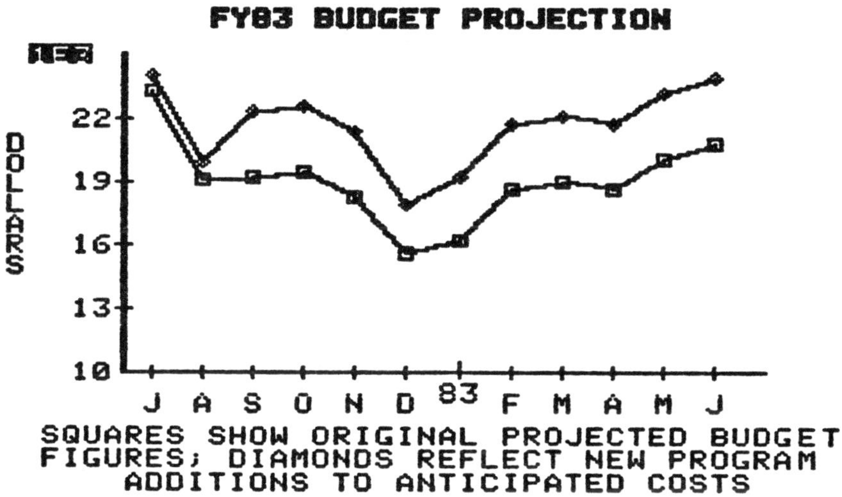

Figure 4-7 New Program Impact: Cumulative Expense Graph

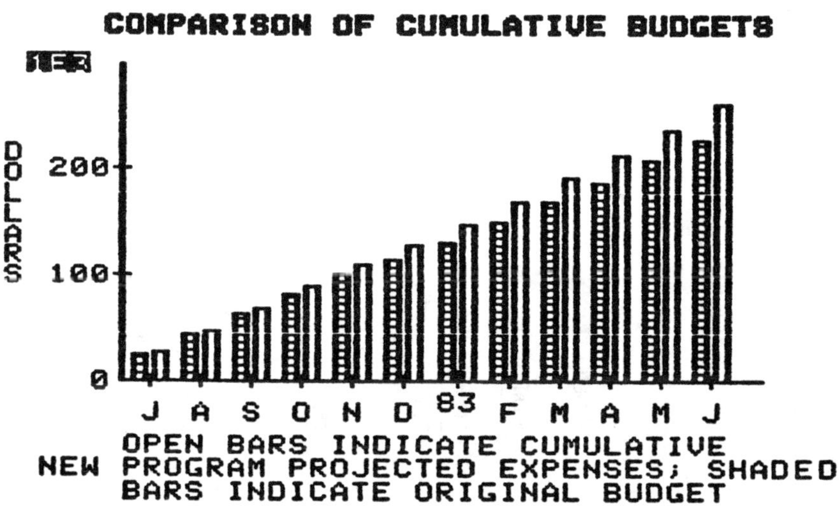

Exhibit 4-35 Budget Projection: New Program

HOSPITAL OPERATIONS
BUDGET PROJECTION FOR FISCAL YEAR:
FOR ACCOUNT NUMBER: 198765
ACCOUNT NAME: TWO WEST OPERATIONS

	JULY	AUG	SEPT	OCT	NOV	DEC	JAN	FEB	MAR	APR	MAY	JUN	TOTAL
BUDGETED PT. DAY	678	699	822	866	809	556	642	798	852	840	897	908	9367

STRAIGHT LINE EXPENSES

EXPENSE CLASS	JULY	AUG	SEPT	OCT	NOV	DEC	JAN	FEB	MAR	APR	MAY	JUN	TOTAL
PROF. AND ADMIN.	2655	2655	2655	2655	2655	2655	2655	2655	2655	2655	2655	2655	31860
SICK/VAC	335	335	335	335	335	335	335	335	335	335	335	335	4020
TOTAL	2990	2990	2990	2990	2990	2990	2990	2990	2990	2990	2990	2990	35880
AFSCME	4231	4231	4231	4231	4231	4231	4231	4231	4231	4231	4231	4231	50772
SICK/VAC	215	215	215	215	215	215	215	215	215	215	215	215	2580
LONGEVITY	38	38	38	38	38	38	38	38	38	38	38	38	456
TOTAL	4484	4484	4484	4484	4484	4484	4484	4484	4484	4484	4484	4484	53808
OFFICE	1890	1890	1890	1890	1890	1890	1890	1890	1890	1890	1890	1890	22680
SICK/VAC	85	85	85	85	85	85	85	85	85	85	85	85	1020
TOTAL	1975	1975	1975	1975	1975	1975	1975	1975	1975	1975	1975	1975	23700
OTHER PAY	145	145	145	145	145	145	145	145	145	145	145	145	1740
MONTHLY TOTALS	9594	9594	9594	9594	9594	9594	9594	9594	9594	9594	9594	9594	115128

PATIENT DAY RELATED EXPENSES

EXPENSE CLASS	INDEX	JULY	AUG	SEPT	OCT	NOV	DEC	JAN	FEB	MAR	APR	MAY	JUN	TOTAL
GEN & OFFICE	1.2356	838	864	1016	1070	1000	687	793	986	1053	1038	1108	1122	11574
MED/SURG	6.9211	4693	4838	5689	5994	5599	3848	4443	5523	5897	5814	6208	6284	64830
PHARMACY	3.1928	2165	2232	2624	2765	2583	1775	2050	2548	2720	2682	2864	2899	29907
LIN-BED-LAUNDRY	2.7687	1877	1935	2276	2398	2240	1539	1778	2209	2359	2326	2484	2514	25934
MONTHLY TOTALS		9572	9869	11605	12226	11422	7850	9064	11266	12029	11859	12664	12819	132245

SPECIAL SCHEDULE EXPENSES

EXPENSE CLASS	JULY	AUG	SEPT	OCT	NOV	DEC	JAN	FEB	MAR	APR	MAY	JUN	TOTAL
CONTRACT SERV.	256	155	876	456	34	145	321	564	134	55	467	976	4439
POSTAGE	44	34	34	45	23	23	23	44	55	33	44	88	490
TELEPHONE	4533	177	188	166	176	156	176	165	188	156	378	267	6726
FOOD	35	48	47	26	58	36	48	25	18	37	48	154	580
MONTHLY TOTALS	4868	414	1145	693	291	360	568	798	395	281	937	1485	12235
MONTHLY PAYROLL EXP.	9594	9594	9594	9594	9594	9594	9594	9594	9594	9594	9594	9594	115128
MONTHLY COMMODIT EXP.	14440	10283	12750	12917	11713	8210	9632	12064	12424	12140	13601	14304	144480
TOTAL MONTHLY EXP.	24034	19877	22344	22513	21307	17804	19226	21658	22018	21734	23195	23898	259608

TOTAL PAYROLL EXPENSE	115128
TOTAL COMMODITY EXPENSE	144480
TOTAL EXPENSE	259608

Figure 4-8 Cost Center Overall Report: Graphics and Commentary

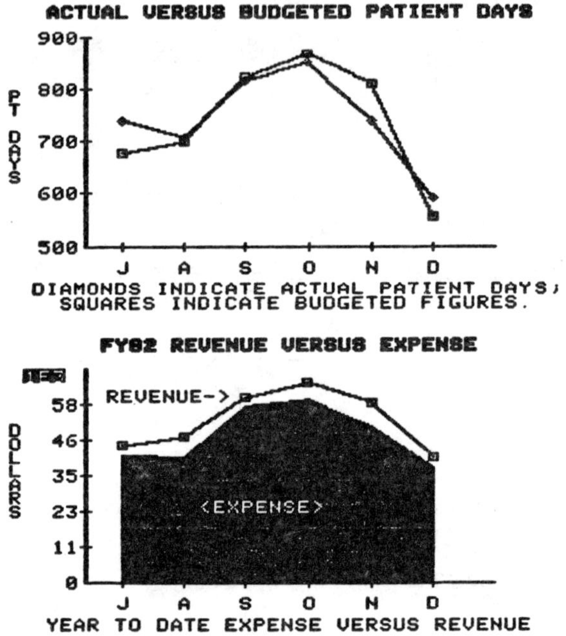

December - Slight increase in patient days (see November comment); expenses were high this month due to charge for past construction costs registered on this cost center.

November - Drop in patient days relative to budget due to medical staff conference during the second week of the month; most patients will be picked up later in the year.

October - Patient days and expense remain close to budget; new program fully implemented, and running as expected.

September - Implementation of new program increases patient days by approximately 165 per month; a corresponding increase is seen in expense. Revenue increased proportionally.

August - Patient days and expense remain close to budget.

July - Patient days up by 10% over budget; due to increased admissions by new medical staff. High expense due primarily to start-up costs of new bed space.

There are, of course, innumerable methods of presenting the data gathered in the reports shown thus far. One very effective format makes use of tables, graphics, and remarks to give an overall report on an account or cost center. Figure 4-8 shows an example of this kind of report.

The format of the report is quite simple; it shows the trends of activity, cost, and revenue for a particular cost center in graphic form at the top of the page. These graphics reflect the most recent data collected for this area.

The second part of the report consists of an accumulation of comments on the tabular and graphic information. Each month's comments include a statement of action taken on a particular issue.

The graphics were prepared using the VisiPlot program and the pictures were saved to a floppy diskette using the appropriate program option. The graphs were then printed (with a dot-matrix printer) onto the upper portion of the paper.

The text remarks are kept in a word processing file. Each month, the new remarks for that month are added in on top of the previous sections. The entire file is printed to allow for easy reference. Note that the remarks are kept brief and to the point to allow for easier reference and a minimum amount of material to look through.

SUMMARY

The microcomputer, along with the canned software that is available, can provide every supervisor, manager, and administrator with an invaluable tool for budget control and forecasting. The ability to use spreadsheet programs alone is worth the price of the machine; in fact, a great many microcomputers have been sold on the strength of this one program.

If the user is able to spend the time, spreadsheet programming can easily be done to allow the microcomputer to help realize the many unfulfilled wishes for reports or analysis that were unattainable because of the length of time it would take to do them by hand.

In the future, integrated system software will provide the ability to produce all of the reports, tables, and graphs in this chapter without having to choose between programs or data formats. In fact, that particular "future" is here today in the Apple Lisa computer, and to a lesser degree in the VisiOn system designed for the IBM Personal Computer, and the Lotus 1-2-3 software program for Apple IIs and the IBM PCs. The cost of these systems is, of course, significantly higher than the cost quoted for the minimum system that produced these reports. The extreme low cost of small microcomputer systems, combined with their extraordinary capabilities, will assure their usefulness in any hospital department.

Chapter 5

Word Processing on a Microcomputer

One of the most useful services that a microcomputer can offer is that of word processing. In the case of micro word processing, it is also one of the most accessible functions offered; some of the simpler programs can be learned within an hour or two. In this chapter, we will explore this application from the standpoints of function and cost and point out some interesting uses for word processing programs.

Most people in business are aware of the concept of word processing and recognize that typing is a form of symbol manipulation at which computers excel. Once a group of symbols is entered into the machine, it need not be entered again for the sake of minor (or even major) correction.

The idea of word processing originated with dedicated minicomputer systems, that is, systems that performed only one function. These systems have advanced during the years that they have been available, both in terms of the low-cost functions offered and the speed and efficiency with which they are performed. However, all word processing systems can be said to consist of the following:

1. Hardware—keyboard, display, microprocessor, internal memory, mass storage, printer, printer interface card
2. Software—text entry and manipulation, file handling, print program

The average business user is accustomed to purchasing a function and is uninterested in the details of how the function is provided. The microcomputer user does not have this luxury; one must pay close attention to all elements of a word processing system. On the other hand, micro word processing systems are extremely flexible, in terms of both software and hardware. This flexibility also extends to the variety of functions available and the cost of the system.

Microcomputers can easily handle the task of word processing, but the user must take care that all of the functions desired are offered by the software and supported by the hardware. At this point in the evolution of the microcomputer, a greater level of expertise is required on the part of the user.

We will now examine word processing systems point by point, comparing dedicated systems with micros, using the list of word processing system elements defined above.

HARDWARE

The Keyboard

The keyboard of a dedicated system typically offers a number of keys not found on a typewriter. These special function keys are linked to the software to allow the user to perform complex tasks with the touch of a single key. The more special keys provided, the more keystrokes saved; however, as the number of keys increases, the amount of skill required on the part of the user increases rapidly. Many professional systems require a month or more of use by the operator before a reasonable level of proficiency is reached.

Most microcomputer keyboards, however, are not noticeably different from those of electric typewriters. The lack of special function keys is a hardware limitation that may be to the user's advantage in the sense that the system has a more familiar initial appearance. Special functions are keyed in one part at a time, with combinations of available keys. It is important to remember that microcomputer hardware and software development was not carried out concurrently with the goal of producing a word processing system. Typically, the provider of the software is not even the same company as the provider of the keyboard.

When purchasing a microcomputer with word processing in mind, it is a good idea to pay close attention to the keyboard, noting the "feel" of the keyboard, the ergonometric features (e.g., sculpted keys and sloped rows). The keyboard is the primary interface with the machine; the major user of the system should be satisfied with the quality of the keyboard provided.

The Display

Most microcomputer word processing systems offer a 24 line by 80 character display; the user need only arrange to have a monitor capable of this sort of display. It is easily handled by a 12 inch standard monitor. Special displays, showing an entire page, are available; however, the high cost of such devices ($1,000–$1,500) has prevented them from coming into widespread use.

It should be noted that not all micros are capable of an 80 column display. The Apple II, for example, has a 40 column display; to produce the 80 character line required for professional quality word processing, it is necessary to buy a special firmware card to plug into the machine. This additional device will add about $125–$300 to the cost of the system. Some microcomputers, particularly the low-end systems, have 24 or 32 character lines whose length typically cannot be altered.

Although the low-end systems (as discussed in Chapter 2) have a line length that is too short for serious word processing, they are ideal for use as a "dumb" terminal connected to a mainframe system; many university mainframes offer excellent word processing software through the use of microcomputers or other computer terminals. Also, the portable micros that offer a short line on a small liquid crystal diode display can be used for text entry at remote locations. For example, bibliographic data can be entered into the machine at the library and subsequently "dumped" into the office computer for final manipulation.

Some micros offer a particular display as a built-in part of the system. The IBM Personal Computer and the TRS80 machines are examples of this sort of system. The prospective buyer should look for the following features in such a system:

1. Is the keyboard attached to the monitor? It may be difficult to tailor the system to your personal comfort.
2. Does the monitor swivel around and tilt up and down? It may be important to your use of the system.
3. Is the display easy to read? It is essential to observe the system in use.

Other micros do not provide a monitor with the system; the Apple II and many low-end systems give the flexibility of purchasing any commercially available display and connecting it to the computer. Given the many options available in display screens, including black and white, green phosphor, and amber screen, many persons prefer to tailor their system to their own preferences.

It is generally not advisable to use a color monitor for word processing. Although the color display is useful for graphics and some software applications, it is not capable of forming the small, precise characters required in a 24 × 80 character text display.

The Microprocessor

As we discussed in Chapter 2, each processor has its own set of instructions. A word processing system written for one microcomputer might not run on another. One example is that of WordStar, a well-known program that runs on the CP/M operating system. This program requires a Z80-based processor; the Apple, to give an example, does not have such a processor.

However, it is possible to adapt the machines that do not come equipped with the required processor by inserting a special card into the body of the machine. This card, of course, will add to the cost of using this particular piece of software.

The Internal Memory

Microcomputer word processing may be broken down into two basic types according to the way they use memory. There are RAM-based systems, which use the internal memory of the machine in text editing; these systems are limited in that they are capable of working with individual documents no larger than the internal memory of the system. This type of system is the fastest to use, because all of the text worked on at a given time is in the machine's solid state memory, which, as we have seen, provides the fastest symbol manipulation.

The second type is the disk-based system, which uses the disk (and its larger memory capacity) in text processing; this system has the advantage of being able to work with larger files. Such a system is slower, however, because of the length of time required to shuttle back and forth to the disk with text. Most dedicated systems have two processors to accomplish the work of editing (paying attention to the user) and filing (putting overflow text on disk and obtaining needed files).

Middle-range machines, those with up to 64K bytes of RAM memory, can handle approximately 30,000 characters of internal document storage; this works out to about 20 double-spaced pages. High-range machines typically have the capacity to store up to 180,000 characters of text.

The mass storage system typically used with a micro is the floppy disk drive. These devices can store from 100,000 to 200,000 characters of text per disk; the disks are, of course, removable so that blank disks may be inserted when one disk becomes full. All microcomputer systems used for business word processing will require at least one disk drive.

Also, some word processing systems offer special features on disk, including automatic "help" key functions to provide an on-line source of information about the program. If you find such features particularly desirable, you may wish to purchase two disk drives; one for the program disk and one for text files.

Another argument in favor of having a two-drive system centers around the copying process used to create additional, or "backup," copies of disks. A two-drive system reads data from one disk and then writes it directly onto the other disk (resident in the other disk drive). However, a one-drive system must read the data, stop, and prompt the user to put in the duplicate disk; the data are then written onto the duplicate. The process must stop again as the computer prompts the user to remove the duplicate and put in the original in order to repeat the process until the duplication process is completed.

The process of backing up important files is not a trivial matter. A disk has an in-use life of about 40 hours; that is to say, 40 hours in which the disk is actually spinning. This relatively short lifetime is of particular concern with disk-based systems. Although a disk costs only about $4, if you consider that a disk that is full of text contains about 20,000 words, written or dictated by a manager and then typed by a secretary, the actual cost of the disk plus files is probably closer to $100. Add to this the intrinsic value of the text (perhaps your only copy of a creative work). A lost or "blown" (ruined) disk is an expensive loss.

An alternative to floppy disks is the hard disk drive, which we mentioned in Chapter 2. These devices have the capability to store from 5 million to 100 million characters per drive; most hard disk drives do not offer removable disks. Most microcomputer word processing systems do not require this amount of storage space.

The Printer

A particularly important peripheral to consider when setting up a microcomputer system to be used with word processing software is the printer. As we have seen, there are two basic printer types to be considered: dot-matrix and fully formed character printers. Dot-matrix printers form characters with groups of dots; the quality of print may vary widely from one printer brand to another. The quality of the letters is determined by the print matrix size, that is, how many dots are used to form each character. For example, most dot-matrix printers initially used a 5×7 array of dots to make letters; most printers did not have true descenders (the portion of a letter that extends below the line, as in the letters y and g). Printers in recent years have been offering 9×11 arrays and better, with true descenders. The technology of these devices has improved considerably in the past several years, both in terms of print quality and price. Dot-matrix printers are now available that provide a print quality virtually indistinguishable from that of the top-quality fully formed character printers.

Dot-matrix printers use several technologies to form the image of letters. The most common type uses an array of pins that strike the ribbon against the paper; this technology is also the cheapest and best developed. A dot-matrix printer technology that will come into increasing prominence is the ink jet printer, which uses a spray of dots to form the letters. The character quality of these printers is excellent. However, the speed is usually slower than that of the pin type (20 characters per second versus 160 cps). Also, the ink jet printers are incapable of producing multiple or carbon copies.

Dot-matrix printers are considerably cheaper than their competition, the fully formed character printers. This variety produces print that is identical to that of a good typewriter; in fact, it does it in an identical way. Most of the letter-quality printers sold are daisy wheel printers; they use a print wheel that has the letters and symbols arranged on a device that looks like a wheel with many spokes. At the end of each spoke is a symbol; when typing, the machine turns the wheel into the appropriate position and a hammer strikes the back of the character, making the impression on the paper. With the exception of the ink jet type, dot-matrix printers are also considerably faster than fully formed character printers within a given price range, typically ten times faster.

Printing text is not the only use for a microcomputer printer. One may also print out graphics created with any of the many programs designed for this purpose. However, most fully formed character printers (in particular the less expensive models) will not print graphics; the dot-matrix printers are ideal for this purpose.

The Printer Interface Card

The printer interface card provides the communication link between the computer and the printer. Rather than go into the technical details of these devices, let us explore several specific functions.

Buffer Interface Card

One capability that you may want to have is that of a buffer. A buffer is basically just a processor and a set of RAM chips providing an additional 16–128 bytes of free memory. This additional space is used solely to store text on its way to the printer. Such a card actually supervises the printing of the document and allows the user to continue working while the printer does its work.

The less expensive fully formed character printers print at an extremely slow rate, typically as slow as 12 characters per second. At that rate, even a single-page memo may take up to five minutes to type. If the printer does not have a buffer, the computer itself must store the text and supervise the printer; while engaged in this task, the computer is not available to the user. To avoid waiting while a document is printed, the buffer-type printer card is used to store text and supervise printing.

Some printers come with an "on-board" buffer; such printers may not require additional buffer space. In fact, if your printer has this capability, it may be a good idea not to have a "smart" interface card; a smart printer and a smart interface card can get into "arguments" that may be difficult to resolve. Be sure the computer dealer assures compatibility.

Graphics Interface Card

Another capability that should be considered is that of a graphics interface card. These cards are used primarily because of their special on-board routines that allow the printing of graphic images on appropriate printers. These cards may also be available with a print buffer.

"Spooling"

As a final option, the prospective user should consider additional software to solve the problem of waiting while text is being printed. Some word processing programs have a capability called "spooling" that will allow the user to interact with the system while the system is supervising the printing of text. Such a program can save on hardware expenses; however, a price is paid in terms of slower response to the needs of the human operator, due to the fact that the computer is dividing its attention between the user and the printer.

SOFTWARE

Why Use the Microcomputer for Word Processing?

There are several advantages to using micros for word processing. The first is cost; word processing can be done for as little as $3,000, including letter-quality printing. Compared with the typical single-station word processor price of $8,000 to $12,000, this represents a tremendous cost savings.

Also, because the functions offered are limited, learning is much easier. Many manufacturers will tell the prospective buyer that it takes up to a month to learn to use their system properly; most micro-based systems can be mastered in an afternoon. This is less threatening to many individuals.

An additional advantage of the low cost is that the capability can be provided to many people in an organization. The ease of formatting, changing, or revising entries makes typing one's own work more attractive.

Perhaps the greatest advantage is that the micro is not a dedicated system; it can still be used for other things. This trend is being introduced by the more expensive dedicated word processor makers; many are now coming out with special filing systems as well as operating systems and program languages.

Choosing a Program

The number of programs that perform word processing on micros has expanded greatly; all of the major microcomputers have several different programs available. The kind of program that is purchased should depend on the uses to which it is to be put. The user should not expect to have all of the advantages that are standard on the most expensive word processors, for example, movement of whole columns to different tab settings and mathematics done on columns of numbers. You may be surprised, however, at the number of sophisticated functions offered by micros.

Some of the unusual additional features include the following:

- glossary function that permits entry of large sections of commonly used text with only a couple of key strokes
- footnoting
- superscript, subscript, special characters
- form letters
- split screen and "windows" to permit examination of widely separated sections of text on a large document
- transfer of paragraphs or pages from one document to another
- global search and replace

The only major difference is the manner in which these functions are performed; typically, the programs are not as comprehensible to the user, because more keystrokes are needed.

AppleWriter

One of the first microcomputer implementations of word processing software was the AppleWriter program, written for the Apple computer. This relatively simple program performed most of the basic functions associated with word processing; the lack of special keys was made up for by using the control and escape keys in conjunction with the regular keys on the keyboard.

Like many of the lower-cost word processors, AppleWriter is almost completely RAM based; the entire program is loaded at the beginning of the session and the program disk may be put away. Later versions of the program offer a "help" function that provides an on-line summary of all of the program commands arranged to aid the individual who is trying to remember how to accomplish an editing or filing task. Because this information is contained in files on the program disk, the disk must be present in the disk drive to make use of the help function. Also, the program works on chunks of text limited by the RAM in the computer.

The program makes use of the full 80 columns of screen; additional formatting is chosen in a print menu by setting margins, headers, footers, page numbers, etc.

AppleWriter is written specifically to run on the Apple II and III; it does not work on other machines and is not portable in that sense. It is, however, a relatively inexpensive program.

WordStar

Another example of a fine word processing program for microcomputers is the WordStar program. WordStar differs from AppleWriter in a number of important ways. First, it is disk based; the WordStar program disk must remain in the disk drive at all times. The reason for this is simple; the program is roughly twice the size of AppleWriter (about 70K bytes). Also, it takes care of the text in a disk-based fashion; a special file is kept by the machine on disk of whatever text is being worked on.

One of the nicest features of the WordStar program is the adjustable help menus that appear as a matter of course on the screen. Instead of just the blank work area with a short data line, the WordStar screen can have most of the basic editing commands written out on the screen. Once the user has memorized the necessary information, these menus may be eliminated, thus freeing up additional screen space for text.

Also, the program shows on the screen exactly what will be printed out on paper, including page breaks. The program also allows for hyphenation, onscreen justification of text, and many other features.

Finally, WordStar is a highly portable program that has been in existence for a number of years and runs on practically every major microcomputer available. If you have learned this system on an IBM PC, for example, and you transfer to another hospital that has an Apple, you can use a version that will be virtually identical to what you already know. This program is, however, probably the most expensive word processing program on the market (but well worth it, according to many users).

MacWrite

The latest entry into the microcomputer word processing market is the MacWrite program written for the Apple Macintosh computer. This program offers many of the features found in the more expensive micro word processing packages, at a significantly lower cost. More importantly, through the use of the Macintosh operating environment, MacWrite reaches a new level of simplicity and ease of use.

We will illustrate the use of the MacWrite program by writing the illustrative material on the Macintosh computer (hereafter referred to as Mac). After turning the Mac on, the user sees the screen shown in Figure 5-1. The screen shows a desktop that is empty except for a disk labeled "Correspondence," and the wastebasket; the presence of the disk indicates that it is currently available in the disk drive. Note also the arrow in the upper left hand corner; this arrow may be moved about the screen with the mouse, a special pointing device described in Chapter 2. The words File, Edit, View, and Special denote special menus that may be "pulled down" with the mouse much as a window shade is closed. Now, we will use the mouse to point to the disk, and open it as if it were a file folder lying on our desk.

Figure 5-2 shows the open file labeled "Correspondence"; in addition, we have opened the nested folder labeled "BOOK STUFF" that contains several items, including a transmission letter to the book editor and the file with the corrections to the book manuscript.

Pointing to the file labeled "Book Notes," we open it and begin word processing. All of the system software is present on the 400K microfloppy, and all of the activity of the system is transparent to the user. No knowledge of disk drives or printers is required on the part of the user.

At the beginning of the session, we set appropriate tabs and margins, and begin typing; Figure 5-3 illustrates this point in the word processing session. Among the other features available by using the mouse to manipulate the items on the ruler are left, right, and center justification, and single, one and one-half, and double spacing.

Figure 5-1 MacWrite Blank Desktop

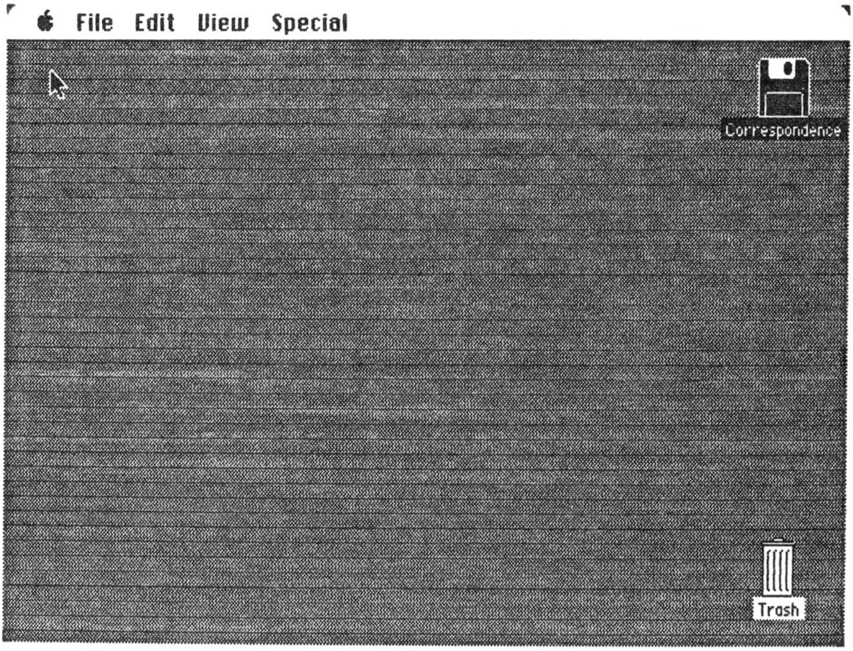

One of the nicest features of the MacWrite program is that it shows the text on the screen exactly as it will be printed. For example, titles or section headings could be in a different type font using enlarged bold print (and underlined), as shown in Figure 5-4. Note that the Style menu has been pulled down, and the bold, underlined, 14 point type has been chosen.

Printing documents is handled in a very simple manner by choosing "Print" from the File menu. All of the choices are made by pointing the mouse at the appropriate "button" and pushing the button on the mouse. The user is prompted to choose the quality of the manuscript, as well as the range of pages to be printed, and the number of copies (see Figure 5-5).

Setting Up the System

When setting up a microcomputer word processing system, the many options provided by software and hardware manufacturers can pose problems. It is important to make sure that the software and the hardware properly complement each other.

Figure 5-2 MacWrite Open File—"Correspondence"

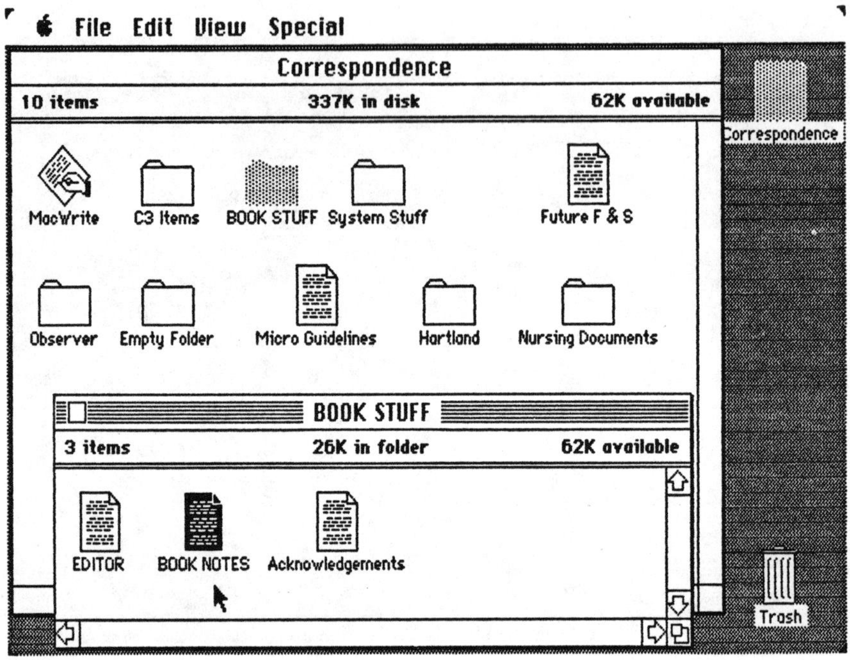

For example, certain functions that may be offered by a software company may not be supported by particular printers. In the case of such special functions as superscripting and subscripting (that is, typing a symbol above or below the line), the software may offer the capability; however, the printer used with the software must have the capability of backing up or going forward one half line to provide these functions. This is not a standard feature on the less expensive printers.

A similar example is that of underlining. Most printers will perform this function but require a special character command to do it. If the software purchased will not allow the user to enter such a command, the underline option cannot be used.

As we have seen, it is also essential that all of the hardware items work together.

Expanding the System

A useful addition to the word processing software is a spelling check program. This piece of software will examine a given file of text and

Figure 5-3 MacWrite Screen: Tabs and Margins Ruler

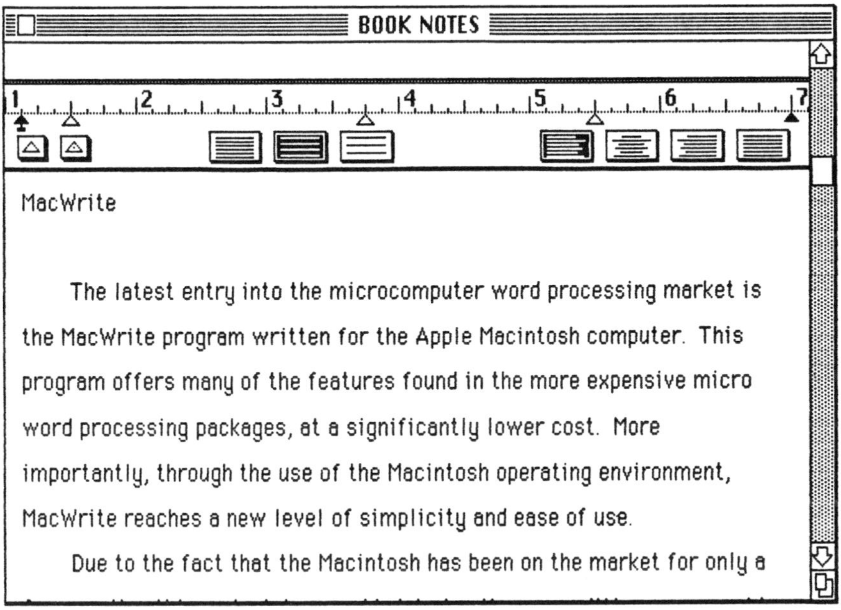

compare each word ("word" is defined as a space followed by one or more characters followed by another space) with the dictionary present on the program disk. If a word is not found, the user is given the following options:

1. Replace the word with a suggested word from the program dictionary.
2. Skip the word and continue searching the text.
3. Add a new word to the speller dictionary.
4. Mark the word for replacement/change later.

The better spelling check programs have the capability of allowing the user to build a dictionary that is specific to the kind of work done. This feature is particularly useful for persons working in a field with a specialized vocabulary.

Note that these programs cannot distinguish between a word that makes sense and one that is spelled correctly. For example, the following sentence would be passed over as correct by a spelling checker: "The first day of the weak is Sunday."

Figure 5-4 MacWrite Screen: Type Styles and Sizes

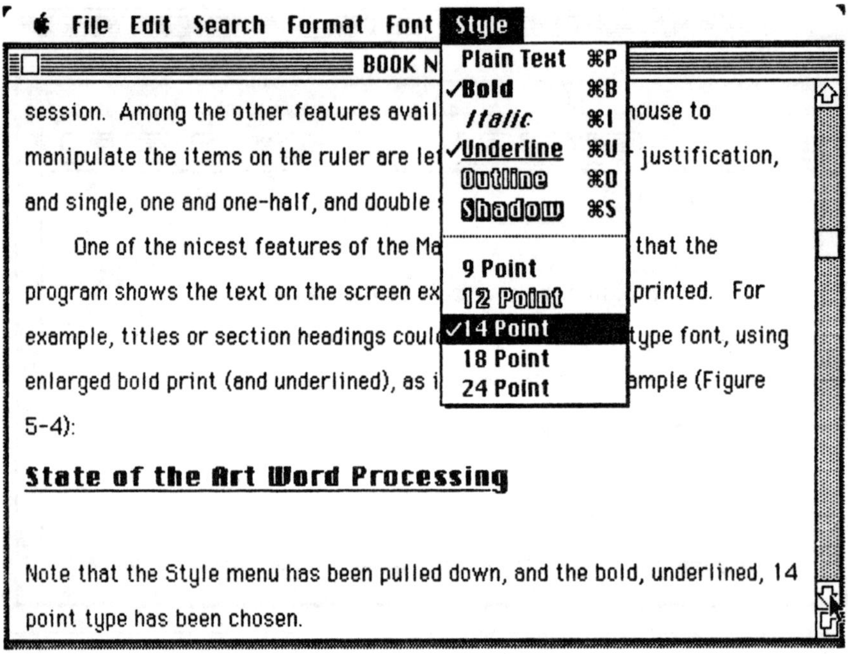

This piece of software does excel in finding the minor errors typical of typed text; transposed characters are easily found and corrected. Because of the time required to load the dictionary with words, however, it may not be practical for the purpose of checking short memoranda; the use of these programs is better suited to the checking of long documents.

Additional capabilities that should be sought in a word processing system are form letter generation, report generation, and label making.

The form letter application involves the printing of a number of copies of a letter, each with an individual name and address. In printing such a letter, it is necessary to build up a data base of names, titles, etc., as well as composing the letter itself. The software retrieves the letter from the disk, adds the name from the disk file, prints the memo, and then continues the process until it runs out of names.

Form letters can be done in the following way, without special software. After entering the memorandum with the first name, send the text to the printer. While waiting for the letter to finish printing, just delete the first name used, and add the new one, and repeat the process.

Although most micro word processing systems do not have mathematical capability, the same functions that provide for a form letter can assist

Figure 5-5 MacWrite Screen: Print Format and Instructions

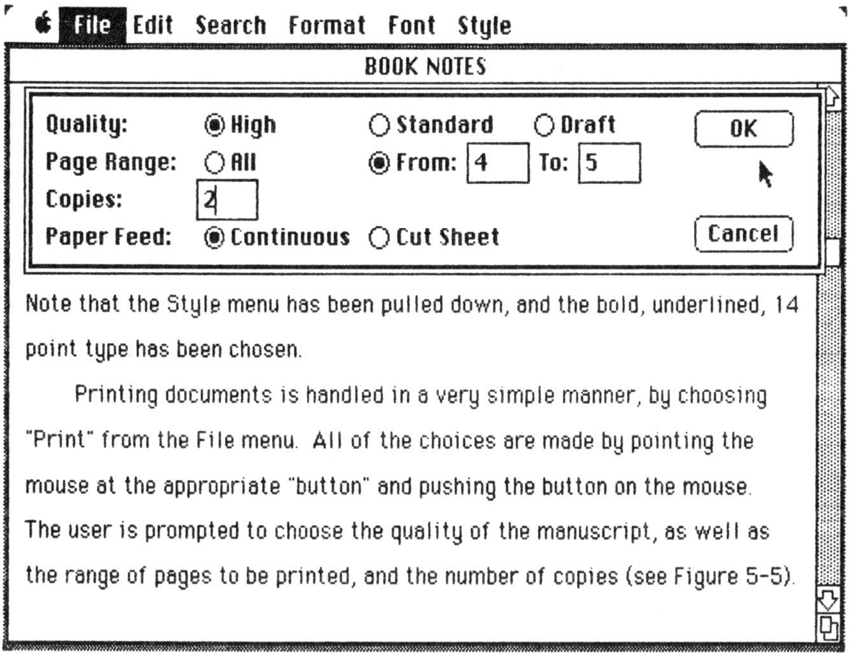

in simple types of report preparation. Many required regular reports contain pieces of information placed in a standard format. A report generator takes bits and pieces from defined text files and inserts them into a report format.

The AppleWriter II program has a particularly flexible Word Processing Language (WPL) that allows the user to program multiple insertions into standard text. Although such an implementation takes longer to master than a simple word processing program, the additional features may be well worth the extra effort.

Other programs, such as WordStar, offer features available at additional cost that provide a mail list type of file manager. This produces files accessible to the word processing program. Having finished the form letter, the mail list file is accessed and the necessary information is placed appropriately in the letter.

CENTRALIZED VERSUS DECENTRALIZED WORD PROCESSING

As we have seen, the cost of a word processing system based on a microcomputer is significantly less than that of dedicated word processors.

Increasingly, offices are examining the service per dollar that can be obtained with micros. A typical example of the dilemma can be seen in the actual case of a manager who was given $15,000 to invest in word processing. He contacted the representative of a well-known manufacturer and received an estimate on a single-station word processor with display, keyboard, processor, disk drives, and a printer; the estimate came to almost $15,000. He then contacted a local computer store and requested a price quote for a word processing system with approximately the same functions; the quote was for $3,000! In other words, he had the choice of obtaining a single dedicated system or five microcomputer-based systems.

Of course, dedicated (or "professional") systems do offer much more elaborate features; the printers on such systems are typically very fast, with features such as boldface, italics, and subscripting. However, the enormous cost differential between the two types of systems is having a profound effect on the word processing industry. In addition, microcomputer software that offers these more advanced features is now available.

Another feature offered by many dedicated systems is a centralized network that allows the users of a system with several machines to share the use of pieces of specialized hardware, such as a fast letter-quality printer. While networking can be done with microcomputers, the concept has not yet been integrated with the word processing software available. It is, of course, a simple matter to place the text to be printed on a floppy disk and then print it out using the micro that is connected to the device required.

LIST MANAGEMENT

An additional use of word processing, beyond the traditional uses of text processing, lies in the area of list management. Although word processing programs do not offer sorting capability, there are a number of uses for word processing systems as simple data base managers.

For example, most managers keep "to do" lists on an ongoing basis. If you are not quite ambitious enough to implement a full-blown problem/suggestion tracking system, you may wish to keep a simple list on your word processing system.

In Exhibit 5-1, a simple "to do" list has been entered in the machine. The advantage of this list is that it can be easily changed and reprinted as time progresses. It should be noted that word processors lack the capability to manipulate the information, in that they cannot provide reports based on the information presented.

Exhibit 5-1 List Management: "To Do" List

```
HOSPITAL OPERATIONS
TASK LIST
NAME:
REVISED:


      TASK                                ASSIGNED COMPLETE  LEAD


Provide room list                          4/1/83  6/1/83    Smith
Coordinate move with housekeeping          4/9/83  4/25/83   Smith
Complete capital equip. request            4/10/83 5/1/83    Smith
```

Besides providing fresh copies of the list on a regular basis, in a relatively painless way, the information is now available in machine-readable form. If a memorandum is being prepared that uses this information (for example, a list of difficulties to a subordinate), the information can be inserted into the memo on the processor.

FACILITIES MANAGEMENT

Word processing programs are also useful in facilities management. Exhibit 5-2 illustrates a page taken from a simple space survey giving the following information: room number, function, major user, square feet,

Exhibit 5-2 Facilities Management: Space Survey

```
HOSPITAL OPERATIONS                                    REVISED:
SPACE INVENTORY                                        RUN DATE:
BUILDING:
AREA:


3459
Patient Room
Nursing
175 sq. ft.
Patient Room Cleaning

3461
Staff Room
Nursing/Clerical
165 sq. ft.
Office Cleaning

3463
Clean Storage
Staff
125 sq. ft.
Ancillary Cleaning

3465M
Maintenance Room
Maintenance
35 sq. ft.
Cleaned by Maintenance

3467
Patient Bath
Staff/Patients
75 sq. ft.
Bathroom/Bath Area Cleaning
```

and housekeeping procedure. The major advantage of keeping such a list in machine-readable form is that it can be readily updated to ensure the continuing accuracy of space information. Also, when providing information regarding services to departments, these lists can be used to make sure that everyone possesses the same information. For example, Exhibit 5-2 shows a space survey that might be given to the housekeeping department to ensure that each room is being cleaned according to the appropriate procedures.

FORMS DEVELOPMENT

Another useful application of word processing programs lies in the area of forms development. It is a relatively simple procedure to enter a form on the computer; with an 80 character line, most forms can be duplicated on the screen. Changes are easily made without having to retype the entire form, thus cutting down on turnaround time between a manager and a secretary. The finished form can be stored on the disk drive and can be called up whenever the formatted item is needed.

If you intend to use the microcomputer for this task, you should ask to see the entire system in action; it is helpful to take along a typical form to enter. Exhibit 5-3 shows a typical example, in this case a project tracking summary.

The extent to which a particular system can reproduce a form is typically limited by the printer; most letter quality printers can only reproduce a report that could have been typed on a single pass on an ordinary electric typewriter. Graphics printers, however, are capable of reproducing forms with boxed-in areas and special logos or other graphics.

POLICY MANUALS AND PHONE DIRECTORIES

Word processing programs are also an ideal choice for policy manuals. Because a policy may change only slightly from year to year, most of the policy is still usable. It is far more time efficient to use a word processing program to make the small changes necessary from year to year. The specialized tab settings and print parameters for these documents can also be stored in special files, cutting down on work and ensuring the uniformity of the documents produced.

In fact, any material that is printed at intervals with only minor corrections can be profitably placed on a micro. Phone directories and administrative organizational charts can also be typed, printed, and stored until the next printing period. Compare the cost and turnaround time of a typical

Exhibit 5-3 Forms Development: Project Tracking Summary

HOSPITAL OPERATIONS REVISED:
TRACKING SUMMARY SHEET RUN DATE:
INDIVIDUAL PROJECT SHEET

DEPARTMENT:
ADMINISTRATOR:

PROJECT NAME: ....

....

....

LEAD: ....

PRIORITY: ....

START DATE: .... COMPLETION DATE: ....

DESCRIPTION: ....

....

....

MATERIALS: ....

....

LABOR: ....

....

....

SPECIAL SERVICES: ....

....

....

RELATED WORK ORDERS: ....

....

type-set hospital phone directory with the simplicity of a constantly updated text in a word processing system. A new directory can be easily and cheaply printed semiannually; given the frequency of facility and organizational change in hospitals today, such a level of response is often needed.

WORD PROCESSING IN THE MEDICAL RECORDS DEPARTMENT

Medical records departments have employed varying levels of sophistication in word processing systems for a number of years. Beginning with typewriters that store information on magnetic tape or cards, the technology has proceeded through the development of internal memory storage to the use of video display, full edit capabilities, and other powerful features.

The decision to use state-of-the-art word processing is usually rooted in the desire or need to correct one or several major problems. These problems are typically related to less than satisfactory quality, timeliness, productivity, or cost of medical record reports. Many hospitals may be interested in eliminating unnecessary costs, increasing productivity, reducing or controlling backlogs, or cutting down turnaround time. Or, there may be a desire to eliminate dependency on outside transcription services or to increase capacity. All of these efforts toward improvement carry with them the need to maintain or improve the quality of reports.

It is well to remember that inadequate medical record report production and distribution may be related to quality of patient care. It is most certainly linked to physician and patient satisfaction as well as to the hospital's ability to bill its accounts.

State-of-the-art word processing systems offer many features that support the above goals. These include text editing capabilities, video display, glossary programs that can be used to store preestablished information such as names and addresses, phrases, or even entire reports (e.g., negative radiology reports), user prompts, shared logic, automatic pagination and footnoting placement, and word wraparound. Word wraparound permits typists to type continuously without worrying about carriage returns. Another valuable feature is simultaneous input and output, which allows the typist to key in new or revised information at the same time previously entered reports are being automatically printed.

If a medical records department cannot afford to acquire state-of-the-art word processing equipment, using microcomputers at much lower cost may be a reasonable alternative in some cases; this would be particularly true in cases where programming and computing capabilities are also desired.

Typically, the medical records department transcribes reports such as discharge summaries, history and physical reports, surgical operation reports, consultations, and progress notes. Other documents not as likely to be produced in the medical records department are pathology reports, radiology reports, EEG and EKG reports, and letters to referring physicians. It is often beneficial to centralize these transcription activities under one service, the medical records department being the one of choice because it usually has people with the most training in managing large-scale transcription activities.

Repetitious Identifying Data

Among the most frequently used features of word processing equipment are those that save the most time and effort on the part of the transcriptionist. Repetitious identifying information such as patient's name, address, location, number, and dates of service all need to be keyed into the processor only once. This information can then be automatically repeated on each successive page of a report, if desired. The automatic entry of captions such as "Chief Complaint," "Review of Systems," "Diagnosis," and "Discharge Status" can also save substantial amounts of time by eliminating large numbers of keystrokes. User prompts that request insertion of specific types of information assist the transcriptionist in the production of more complete and accurate reports.

Automatic page formatting and pagination are also time savers and guarantee uniformly produced reports as well. The use of video display allows the transcriptionist to see exactly what will be printed and to make necessary revisions prior to printing. This saves both time and paper. The video display also enables the typist to exert control over the keyed information in much more powerful ways than typing on paper could ever do. Text can be edited quite easily by simply using the command keys to move the cursor to the desired part of the text, inserting or deleting text, or moving text from one place to another.

Glossary Programs and Spelling Dictionaries

Two of the most advanced and intriguing features recently introduced are glossary programs and spelling dictionaries. Glossary programs have been used to produce routine reports for specialties such as radiology. They have great applicability in the production of radiology reports because the findings of radiological examinations are most often either negative or normal. The glossary programs offer transcriptionists the opportunity to select from a number of preestablished formats and stored text, both for general medical reports (i.e., discharge summaries, history and physical examination reports, consultation reports, and reports of surgical operations) and the more specialized reports related to medical disciplines such as radiology.

To begin, a base of phrases or paragraphs is created. The transcriptionist selects the desired format and/or stored text from a video display and causes it to be inserted into the report being produced by means of a command key or word. The material is automatically inserted. In some instances, the entire body of a report is stored and automatically produced. The transcriptionist is prompted by the system to enter any required patient identification information or dates, etc. The system then inserts appropriate headings, page numbers, and, if programmed, a physician name and signature line. The operator then instructs the system by means of special command keys, letters, or words to send the report electronically to the printer, where it is printed in finished form.

The system may also employ a dictionary or lexicon of correct spellings. These can be entered by the operator individually or purchased as a package of terms. Commercially produced spelling dictionaries are available to be "plugged" into the system. These dictionaries often contain thousands of words and can be general in nature or tailored to special fields such as medicine or law. The dictionary created by the operator would take time to produce but could be closely tailored to the specific transcription task at hand. These dictionary systems work by automatically checking each word as it is keyed into the system against a spelling "authority list." In cases where there appears to be a misspelled word (the keyed word does not match the authority), the word is highlighted in some way. The operator can then either correct the original spelling or override the system. The operator would override in cases where there might be more than one correct spelling for a word or where a special spelling is desired.

Productivity Improvements

Dedicated word processing systems are marketed by companies that claim productivity improvements of 40 or 50 percent. However, these claims appear to be somewhat exaggerated. The reason they may seem so high is that they may consider as production total revisions of previously entered material. While it might be quite reasonable to do this, for example, if previous practice required total retyping of a document on a standard typewriter, in many cases the entire report would not necessarily have been retyped. Only the words to be revised might have been changed. Counting as production an entire document of many pages when only a small number of words or letters has been changed is only appropriate if the entire document would have had to be redone in any case. Most medical transcription services are not involved in manuscript production. Thus, the opportunity to reproduce entire documents, whether or not this would have been done in the first place, results in the opportunity to inflate production figures and thereby mask reality.

Nevertheless, productivity gains in the 20–30 percent range are quite achievable in a medical records setting, and gains of that magnitude warrant the acquisition of word processing equipment in virtually any hospital. Depending on the size of one's operation, the payback would be in the two- to three-year range with modest productivity gains. If the nature of documents was such that productivity gains in the 40 to 50 percent range were achievable, the payback period would be one to two years. These estimates are predicated on equipping a shared logic four-station system costing about $50,000 at 1984 prices.

The cost of four microcomputers with word processing programs of high quality would run in the $15,000–$20,000 range. The payback period for this type of setup could easily be less than one year.

Radiology Transcription

The radiology function may provide one of the best potential areas for cost reduction through the merging of files of information. Using the system's glossary programs, preestablished text can be entered into storage for large numbers of reports of "normal" findings. In these cases, the glossary feature goes beyond the insertion of headings, captions, and other prompts and produces paragraphs or the entire text of the reports automatically. The transcriptionist simply enters the patient's identifying information and the date. Since most radiology reports indicate normal findings, this feature can prove to be of great benefit.

Histories and Examination Reports

Another intriguing use of word processors in the medical records setting is the application of glossary programs to the production of history and physical examination reports. Many efforts have been made to establish this type of system, going back to the use of magnetic tape or card typewriters. The advent of sophisticated word processors offers much more promise than ever before in this regard, short of the use of large and expensive computer systems to do the same job.

Systems such as the Apple Lisa may come to be viewed as a breakthrough in this regard because of their user friendliness, great capacity, and reasonable cost. In this type of system, the user precodes a number of phrases, sentences, and/or paragraphs to selected key commands. The physician, while performing the exam, or shortly after, uses a checklist to indicate the phrase or words to be used to describe his or her findings. If no words or phrases have been established to enter a particular finding, the physician overrides by writing the desired information. The transcriptionist keys information on the checklist using the command codes or physician override information, thus saving large numbers of keystrokes. The system illustrated in Exhibit 5-4 would require a large and sophisticated word processing or microcomputer setup; a simple 64K processor could not do such a large job. The report generated by this approach is shown in Exhibit 5-5.

Essentially, the system is a broader application of the radiology system. The greater generality of the history requires greater flexibility of operation. The greatest applicability of the history system may, therefore, be found in the clinic or private practice setting where controls exist emanating from individual physicians. The limitations of such systems lie in the need to tailor the precoded information to individual subspecialties or individual habits. While the ophthalmologist will no doubt spend extensive time (and words) on the EYES section of the exam, the neurologist would be more concerned with the NEUROPSYCHIATRIC section. Many medical subspecialties have developed systems tailored to their needs, whether manual or automated. These systems should provide for lengthy precoded documentation.

The same approach could be taken for the physical exam report, discharge summary, and other reports. The degree of sophistication depends on the need and system size. Care should be taken to ensure that any medical information system is developed using the standards of the Joint Commission on Accreditation of Hospitals.

System Control

Two caveats are in order when considering the acquisition of word processing equipment. First, it is essential that reasonable, quantifiable objectives be set and that progress be measured against those goals. The investment in word processing is not minor, and the return on investment will be achieved only if controls are in place and monitored to ensure the maintenance of productivity gains over time. Second, the use of word processing capabilities and equipment should be controlled by placing restrictions on the type of work to be done. Opening the system to unsolicited (often extraneous) use, such as the dumping of routine correspondence that should be processed elsewhere, invites losses in productivity. Constant surveillance and attention to overall goals are essential. With these cautions in mind, a hospital can move rapidly to the achievement of extensive medical record word processing improvements.

Exhibit 5-4 Glossary Program: Patient History Checklist

PATIENT NAME____________________
HISTORY CHECKLIST RECORD NO____________________
DATE____________________

HISTORY

CHIEF COMPLAINT (25 WORD LIMIT):
HISTORY OF PRESENT ILLNESS (75 WORD LIMIT):
HISTORY OF PAST ILLNESSES:
P1 CHILDHOOD:
P2 ADULT:
P3 INJURIES:
P4 OPERATIONS:
FAMILY HISTORY:
F1 FATHER 1-ALIVE 2-DECEASED AGE:
MEDICAL HISTORY:
F2 MOTHER 1-ALIVE 2-DECEASED AGE:
MEDICAL HISTORY:
S1 SIBLING #1 SEX: M–F 1-ALIVE 2-DECEASED AGE:
MEDICAL HISTORY:
S2 SIBLING #2 SEX: M–F 1-ALIVE 2-DECEASED AGE:
MEDICAL HISTORY:
S3 SIBLING #3 SEX: M–F 1-ALIVE 2-DECEASED AGE:
MEDICAL HISTORY:
S4 SIBLING #4 SEX: M–F 1-ALIVE 2-DECEASED AGE:
MEDICAL HISTORY:
S5 OTHER:
SOCIAL HISTORY:
SH1 MARRIED
SH2 SINGLE
SH3 CHILDREN NO:
SH4 DOES NOT SMOKE
SH5 SMOKES PACKS PER DAY:
SH6 DOES NOT DRINK
SH7 DRINKS SOCIALLY ONLY
SH8 DRINKS OZ. PER DAY
SH9 DRUGS 1-YES 2-NO NOTE:
SH0 OCCUPATION (LIMIT 20 LETTERS):
SYSTEMIC REVIEW:
GENERAL:
G1 FEVER 1-NO 2-YES
G2 WEIGHT 1-NO CHANGE 2-LOSS 3-GAIN LBS: CURRENT:
G3 INSOMNIA 1-NO 2-YES DURATION:
G4 OTHER:
SKIN:
SK1 RASHES 1-NO 2-YES
SK2 PRURITIS 1-NO 2-YES
SK3 OTHER:

Exhibit 5-4 continued

HEAD:
H1 HEADACHE 1-NO 2-YES
H2 DESCRIPTION:
H3 OTHER:
EYES:
E1 GLASSES 1-NO 2-YES 3-READING GLASSES ONLY
E2 GLASSES LAST CHANGED:
E3 SCOTOMA 1-NO 2-YES
E4 DIPLOPIA 1-NO 2-YES
E5 COLOR BLINDNESS
E6 PAIN 1-NO 2-YES
E7 LID SWELLING 1-NO 2-YES
E8 INFLAMMATION 1-NO 2-YES
E9 OTHER:
EARS:
EA1 HEARING (DESCRIBE):
EA2 PAIN 1-NO 2-YES DESCRIBE:
EA3 DISCHARGE 1-NO 2-YES DESCRIBE:
EA4 POSTAURICULAR PAIN 1-NO 2-YES
EA5 POUNDING 1-NO 2-YES DESCRIBE:
EA6 TINNITIS 1-NO 2-YES DESCRIBE:
EA7 OTHER:
NOSE:
N1 SENSE OF SMELL (DESCRIBE):
N2 OBSTRUCTION 1-NO 2-YES
N3 EPISTAXIS 1-NO 2-YES
N4 OTHER:
THROAT:
T1 SORE THROAT 1-NO 2-YES FREQUENCY:
T2 OTHER
NECK:
NE1 NO MASSES
NE2 OTHER (DESCRIBE):
RESPIRATORY:
R1 PLEURISY 1-NO 2-YES
R2 HEMOPTYSIS 1-NO 2-YES
R3 OTHER:
CARDIOVASCULAR:
C1 PRECORDIAL PAIN 1-NO 2-YES
C2 DYSPNEA 1-NO 2-YES
C3 ORTHOPNEA 1-NO 2-YES
C4 NIGHT DYSPNEA 1-NO 2-YES
C5 PEDAL EDEMA 1-NO 2-YES
C6 HYPERTENSION HX 1-NO 2-YES
C7 OTHER:
GASTROINTESTINAL:
GI1 APPETITE (DESCRIBE):
GI2 JAUNDICE 1-NO 2-YES

Exhibit 5-4 continued

GI3 DIARRHEA 1-NO 2-YES
GI4 INDIGESTION 1-NO 2-YES
GI5 OTHER:
GENITOURINARY:
GN1 DYSURIA 1-NO 2-YES
GN2 BURNING 1-NO 2-YES
GN3 INCONTINENCE 1-NO 2-YES
GN4 HX OF KIDNEY DISEASE 1-NO 2-YES
GN5 OTHER:
GYNECOLOGICAL:
GY1 NOT APPLICABLE
GY2 AGE AT MENARCHE:
GY3 CURRENT CYCLE EVERY DAYS; DURATION:
GY4 DYSMENORRHEA: 1-NO 2-YES
GY5 GRAVIDA:
GY6 MENOPAUSE AT AGE:
GY7 LEUCORRHEA 1-NO 2-YES
GY8 OTHER:
MUSCULOSKELETAL:
MU1 DESCRIBE:
MU2 NO PRESENT PROBLEMS:
NEUROPSYCHIATRIC:
NU1 DESCRIBE:
NU2 NO PRESENT PROBLEMS:
CURRENT MEDICATIONS:
CM1 LIST:
DATE REPORT COMPLETED:
DATE TRANSCRIBED:

WORD PROCESSING POTENTIAL

It is difficult to predict the effect that very low-cost word processing ($2,500 or less per station) will have on the way that business is done in hospitals. At the very least, it will extend this capability to many persons whose status in the hospital hierarchy does not warrant the expenditure of $12,000 to $20,000 for a word processing system. That is, the ability to easily modify and improve memoranda and reports, as well as to pursue the more creative uses mentioned above, will now be within the reach of supervisors and managers as well as top-level administrators.

Also, the mere fact that the service can be provided on a machine that is perhaps only twice as expensive as a high quality electric typewriter, a machine that can offer so much more than a typewriter can, will direct many buyers toward the purchase of a microcomputer.

Exhibit 5-5 Glossary Program: Patient History Report

HISTORY REPORT

PATIENT NAME Doe, John
RECORD NUMBER 123456789
DATE Sept. 12, 1983

CHIEF COMPLAINT: "Seizures" of six month duration

HISTORY OF PRESENT ILLNESS: About six months ago began to have headaches, confined to right temporal area. Increased intensity over past month. Decreased memory noted. No speech dysfunction. Some petit mal-type seizures. Increased in frequency over past three weeks, several per day. No paralysis, loss of consciousness or walking uncoordination. No parasthesia in lower extremities.

HISTORY OF PAST ILLNESSES: Childhood diseases: measles, mumps. No adult diseases. No operations. Injuries: Fractured left knee in 1969, hospitalized. No allergies.

FAMILY HISTORY: Father alive, age 71. Diabetic. Mother alive, age 67. Hypertensive, history of breast cancer, for which operated in 1969, with no known recurrence. No siblings. No cardiac disease, mental illness, renal disease, seizure disorders, asthma or tuberculosis in family history.

SOCIAL HISTORY: Married, 3 children. Non-smoker, non-drinker, no drug use. Employed as truck driver.

SYSTEMIC REVIEW:
General: No fever, weight loss or insomnia.
Skin: No rashes or pruritis.
Head: See history of present illness.
Eyes: Wears glasses for reading. Last change: February 1981. No scotoma, no diplopia, no color blindness, no pain, no swelling, no inflammation.
Ears: Hearing excellent. No pain, no discharge, no postauricular pain. Some ear pounding, right ear after headaches. No tinnitis.
Nose: Good sense of smell. No obstruction. Epistaxis. Occasionally, brief duration.
Throat: No sore throat.
Neck: No masses.
Respiratory: No pleurisy, no hemoptysis.
Cardiovascular: No dyspnea, no precordial pain, no orthopnea, no pedal edema, no night dyspnea. No history of hypertension.
Gastrointestinal: Good appetite, no jaundice, no diarrhea, no indigestion.
Genitourinary: No dysuria, no burning, no incontinence, no history of kidney disease.
Gynecological: Not applicable.
Musculoskeletal: Diagnosed as having "bursitis" of left shoulder, about 10 years ago. Takes salicylates.
Neuropsychiatric: See history of present illness.

CURRENT MEDICATIONS: Salicylates.

REPORTED: September 13, 1983
TRANSCRIBED: September 14, 1983

In summary, microcomputers offer health care institutions the ability to perform basic word processing as well as a number of other more inventive applications, such as:

- preparation of personnel paperwork, with the potential to link information generated on the micro to central personnel files automatically
- creation and management of "lists," such as "things to do" lists, space inventories, project tracking, donor lists, lists of regulatory citations and corrective actions, problem lists, quality assurance activity lists, and telephone directories, to name a few
- maintenance of standard document formats for such things as meeting agendas, committee membership lists, policy and procedure manuals, contracts and general correspondence
- complete maintenance of policy and procedure manuals, including distribution lists (word processing offers the opportunity for considerable savings of time and money in this regard)
- transcription of standard medical and nonmedical reports
- composition of patient menus for mass production
- creation and maintenance of repetitive work schedules, task lists, and inventory sheets
- creation and editing of articles and books (such as this one)

These are just a few of the types of applications that can be easily accomplished on a microcomputer with word processing capability. Innovative supervisors and managers will no doubt create many other imaginative uses.

Chapter 6

Data Base Management with Microcomputers

If there is any single task that is common to all computer programs, it would be that of data base management (DBM). Simply stated, DBM is the process by which information is stored and retrieved so that it may be used. In this chapter, we will explore the process of data base management as it is performed by microcomputers. A number of applications will be considered, using commercially available programs as well as some custom software.

Though all computer programs make use of the data base management process, the manner in which it is performed varies from one computer system to another. The first step in performing this function involves defining the data to be stored and the manner in which it will be stored. Let us take as a practical example the case of a space inventory program in which we want to keep track of all of the rooms in a facility, including information related to room number, square feet, function of the space, etc.

FIELDS, RECORDS, AND FILES

The individual pieces of data (e.g., a room number, or the square footage associated with that room number) may be placed in fields within a larger unit called a record. A record, in the case of our example, might therefore consist of all of the individual pieces of data associated with a particular room. All of the records for a particular patient floor might be combined into a larger unit called a file.

Thus, we might define a certain file called, let us say, "6 West," and that file would consist of perhaps 70 records. The first record would consist of all of the data to be kept on Room 601, and would therefore contain, for example, four fields of data in order to keep track of the room number, square feet, function, and the number of workstations.

The file would, therefore, look like this:

File "6 West"
  Record 1
    Field 1
    Field 2
    Field 3
    Field 4
  Record 2
    Field 1
    Field 2
    and so on.

STORING INFORMATION

There are two major formats for storing information, each with its own advantages. The first to be considered is called a sequential file. In a sequential file, all of the data fields are butted directly up against each other, so that they would look something like this on the disk drive:

```
R/601/150/Nurse Station/6/R/602/110/Clean Storage/0/R/
603/180/Semi-Private/2/ and so on.
```

In the second type of storage, called random access files, each record, and each data field within the record, has a certain defined length. The same file would look like this:

```
R/601   /150   /Nurse Station    /6 /R/602   /110   /
Clean Storage    /0 /R/603   /180   /Semi-Private     /
2 /
```

In the sequential file, the three records shown take up 58 characters on the disk. The random access file takes up 105 characters of space to save the same information. From the standpoint of saving storage space, a sequential file is clearly the most economical.

However, there is a problem with sequential files. In order to make use of the information, the computer must go to the disk, find the record needed, and read it into its internal RAM memory. The only way for the computer to find information in a sequential file is to read through every record, starting with the first one, until it finds the record requested. The sequential storage method can be likened to the way that songs are stored on a tape recorder; if you want to listen to the third song, you have to go through the first and the second.

Random access files, on the other hand, can be accessed at random (hence the name) for the very reason that all of the files have exactly the same length. Given the starting point of the file on the disk, the computer can calculate the position of the third record, and go there directly. Random access filing systems are therefore many times faster in operation and are preferred by many programmers.

SORTING DATA

Having determined the most efficient method of storing and retrieving the data, the next step is to find out the kind of manipulation that will be needed to produce reports from the data. Typically, this involves sorting the data according to some particular criterion or set of criteria.

There are many ways of sorting data. The most simple kind of sort is called a bubble sort.

Consider the following series of numbers:

10 7 9 6 11

Let us suppose we would like these numbers in order from greatest to least. All sorting methods involve two distinct processes: comparing one item with another and switching the position of items based on the comparisons.

In our example, the machine would start by comparing the first item with the second and determining if item 1 was greater than item 2. Since it is, it would then compare item 1 with item 3, and so on. Finally, it would compare item 1 with item 5 and find that item 5 is greater. The computer would then switch item 1 with item 5, so the new array would look like this:

11 7 9 6 10

The computer would then start with item 2 and compare it with the items following it in the array. A number of such "passes" would be made through the data until item 4 was compared with item 5 and the largest numbers floated to the top (hence the name—bubble sort). The string would then be ordered from greatest to least, as we requested.

In a computer, each operation takes a little bit of time to perform. Every time a comparison is made, or a switch is performed, a small amount of time is taken. A computer could perform the above sort on a five-item array in less than a second. However, as the number of items in the array increases, the number of necessary operations increases dramatically. A useful criterion to keep in mind when purchasing a DBM program is the length of time that the program takes to sort an array of data elements, if such a figure is available.

Getting back to our example, let us suppose we now want to produce a list of rooms sorted in terms of square feet, largest to smallest. The program would obtain the necessary data, sort the array, and produce the needed report. Other kinds of sorting that might be done would be found in a report asking for all of the patient rooms in a given file. Or, the user may want a list of all rooms larger than 100 square feet.

An additional form of sorting that can be very useful allows the user to define a number of characteristics to search for in a file of particular records. For example, the user may want a list of all offices with greater than 100 square feet of space.

REPORT GENERATION

The final capability of DBM programs that we will look at in general outline is called the report generator. Having stored the data, retrieved it, and sorted it, the program must now print it on paper. Most DBM programs allow the user some flexibility in designing reports, which would typically be in a columnar format. Our space inventory example would look like this:

Room Number	Function	Square Feet	Workstations
601	Nursing Station	150	6
602	Clean Storage	110	0
603	Semi-Private	180	2

MEMORY

The primary limitation to effective data base management with microcomputers has to do with the mass storage device used to handle the stored information.

As we stated in Chapter 2, there are two major forms of memory used by a micro. The first, electronic random access memory (RAM), is very fast to use but limited in quantity. Also, this form of memory is volatile, that is, it does not retain the information stored in it when the power is turned off. The second, "mass memory," may employ a floppy disk or a hard disk on which the information is permanently kept.

Three characteristics of disk drives are of major importance in determining the efficiency of a data base management system. The first is the speed with which the computer can find the information stored (access time). The second is the rate at which the data are copied from the disk into the computer's internal memory for manipulation (transfer rate). The final major characteristic is the size of the disk drive unit, that is, how much data can be stored per unit.

Access time is important because in many data base management tasks the data are not read off as a whole (i.e., records 1 through 100 sequentially) but rather are accessed randomly, as each record is needed. Recall that because the internal memory of the computer is limited in a microcomputer, as few records are present in RAM memory as possible.

The data transfer rate is also vital to the process in terms of the speed with which a given task will be accomplished. We have noted that the transfer rate of a hard disk may be ten times faster than that of a floppy disk drive. If, for example, a task involves the examination and manipulation of a great many records, using a hard disk may mean the difference between waiting ten minutes for a result versus an hour or more with floppies.

Also, because hard disks may store from 30 to 100 times as much information per unit, it is much more convenient to manipulate large files with a hard disk. For example, a file of 1,000 records, each of which consists of 1,000 characters of information, would take up about 1,000,000 bytes on the disk. Because hard disks could easily handle a file of this size, the manipulation could proceed without human attention. However, because most floppy disks contain only about 150,000 bytes of space, the 1,000 record file would be spread out over several diskettes. The manipulation of the file would require that someone be present to insert and remove disks from the floppy disk drive.

CHOOSING A DBM PROGRAM

There are a number of commercially available programs that perform generalized data base management functions. That is, they are not designed to keep track of specific data but may be used for a wide variety of tasks.

These programs vary in complexity from emulating a small index file card system (that is, small records that could be sorted on a number of different fields) to programs capable of tracking tens of thousands of large records and producing detailed reports automatically.

When deciding which is the best DBM system for your use, the following questions should be considered:

1. Who will use the program? Will it be used by novices with little training or by persons with some degree of computer expertise?
2. How many data will be kept, in terms of the total number of bytes (or characters of text)?
3. What kind of manipulation is required?
4. What kind of report will be needed?

In considering who will use the system, it should be noted that the greater the capability of a given system, the more complex it will be to operate. Some of the more powerful programs may take your staff weeks to master. That is, they must learn the process by which files are set up and reports are prepared. However, once a data file has been set up, and the parameters of the report to be produced have been defined, a less expert person can be trained to operate the system for the tasks of data entry and report production.

The amount of data to be stored is important in several respects. As we have seen, if very large amounts of data are kept (in excess of one million bytes), a hard disk system becomes very attractive. Also, most programs have inherent limits to the number of records that can be handled.

Manipulation will typically take the following forms:

- sort on one or more fields of data
- combine fields of data mathematically (e.g., add all of the square footages in our previous example to obtain a total by unit)
- statistical analysis of data produced

Clearly, the more complex the manipulation, the more closely the DBM program comes to resemble electronic spreadsheet programs, in that fields of data are combined, percentages taken, etc., over a number of records (or rows on a spreadsheet). The difference is that the DBM program will not show what it has in a columnar format on the screen.

The final item, the reports to be printed, should be examined in terms of how many characters should be placed on a line. For instance, most printers using 8½ × 11 paper can only print, at most, 132 characters on a line. A report requiring more would need a special wide-bed printer.

The use of the system as described in Chapter 3 on microcomputers in the hospital environment should be carefully considered, keeping in mind the pitfalls of doing large-scale programming and data collection.

SPECIAL PURCHASE TRACKING

In the example that follows, the micro will be used in a special purchase tracking system. This application could easily be implemented (given sufficient disk storage space) to handle the load from a small hospital or a major department.

The first step is to set up the record for the purchase order information. Exhibit 6-1 illustrates a sample record. The data tracked include all purchasing information for an individual item as well as the persons responsible for the ordering and stocking of the item. Indicating the purpose of the item and its importance gives the user a perspective on each item. The inclusion of an alternate source (more than one alternative can, of course, be given) allows the user to make use of competition to keep prices as low as possible and to maintain an appropriate level of supply.

The next step is to start a separate series of records related to individual orders; the record would contain the following fields:

Item name:
Ordered by (name):
Quantity ordered:
Estimated cost:
Date of order:
Order required by (date):
Requisition number:
Purchase order number:
Order received by firm:
Order shipped by firm:
Items received:
Order cost:

The user would then merely begin entering the necessary data at any point in the fiscal year. This data base has an obvious utility already; by placing all of this information in one place, and printing it out (as is) when needed, much of the paperwork associated with keeping track of orders can be simplified.

Exhibit 6-1 Purchase Order Tracking: Sample Record

PURCHASE ORDER TRACKING

Item Name:

Source Company:

Address:

City:

State:

Zip:

Phone Number:

Sales Representative:

Delivery Lag Time:

Cost per Item:

Shipped Via:

Alternative Source:

Address:

City:

State:

Zip:

Phone Number:

Sales Representative:

Delivery Lag Time:

Cost per Item:

Shipped Via:

Average Order Size:

Average Order Cost:

Purpose of Item:

Relative Importance:

Responsible Manager:

However, this is only the start of the usefulness of having a data base. For example, suppose you wanted to know who had ordered what (and at what cost) over a year's time. With the data base management programs available, the user would have to enter specific sort criteria and all of the relevant information would be printed out, by user, with only the fields needed (item and cost).

Another use of this system would be to produce a report, sorted by vendor, detailing the performance of the vendor with regard to timely delivery of products.

To find out the orders outstanding, just print out all records in which the "date received" is still blank. Orders that are behind the date promised can easily be determined by sorting the appropriate field relative to the present date.

PROJECT TRACKING

The computer-supported tracking system described below is an existing system developed by the authors that can be quite useful in tracking smaller projects. Intended as a personal tracking tool for individual users, it has the capability of tracking up to 100 projects per file. Because of its design and capacity, a separate disk file must be created for each individual user. The program will print all projects in the current file under only one heading.

The program is written in Applesoft BASIC and will run on any Apple II Plus or IIe computer. The program consists of the following components: several computer screen formats that allow the user to interact with the program in order to create, revise, and delete information, and several report formats that allow the user to obtain easy to use information based on what has been entered.

The interactive screens look like this:

```
GENERAL HOSPITAL
PROJECT TRACKING SYSTEM

PLEASE CHOOSE ONE OF THE FOLLOWING:

1. ADD A NEW PROJECT
2. VIEW OR ALTER EXISTING PROJECTS
3. PRINT PROJECT LISTS
4. EXIT THIS PROGRAM
```

By pressing "1" and the "RETURN" key, the user causes the following screen to appear:

```
PROJECT NUMBER:  1.

PROJECT TITLE:   ?. . . . . . . . . . . . . . . . . . . .

STARTING DATE:   ?. . . . . . . . . . . . . . . . . . . .

TARGET DATE:     ?. . . . . . . . . . .

RANK:            ?. . . . . . . . . . .

LEAD:            ?. . . . . . . . . . . . . . . . . . . .

NOTES:
1.     . . . . . . . . . . . . . . . . . . . . . . . . . . . . . . . . . .
2.     . . . . . . . . . . . . . . . . . . . . . . . . . . . . . . . . . .
3.     . . . . . . . . . . . . . . . . . . . . . . . . . . . . . . . . . .
4.     . . . . . . . . . . . . . . . . . . . . . . . . . . . . . . . . . .
5.     . . . . . . . . . . . . . . . . . . . . . . . . . . . . . . . . . .
6.     . . . . . . . . . . . . . . . . . . . . . . . . . . . . . . . . . .

ENTER DATA AS INDICATED BY CURSOR
TO RETURN TO MAIN MENU TYPE 'QUIT'
```

The user is now free to create a project or other item to be tracked by entering the relevant information. The "ENTER" key is pressed after each item on the screen; this moves the cursor to the next item. Once the project is described, the user presses "RETURN" again. This enters the data into disk storage. The same screen reappears; this time it is once again empty. The user now has the opportunity to enter another project or item description. The process may be repeated for up to 100 projects.

When the user has completed entering information on the items to be tracked, the work "QUIT" is typed. This returns the user to the MAIN MENU. If the user chooses to view or revise information on a given project or item, the number "2" is typed. The program has loaded the information on each project into memory with the exception of the NOTES. The program now displays the project titles:

```
PROJECT LISTING BY TITLE

1.   MOVE DINING ROOM EQUIPMENT
2.   INSTALL NEW DISCHARGE PLANNING SYS
3.   CREATE POSTER FOR MARKETING
4.   CHANGE ALL LIGHTING - 3W
5.   IMPLEMENT SALARY PROGRAM
6.   PROCURE FLOOR MATS
7.   CLEAN SCREENS

A)DD, D)ELETE, C)HANGE, M)ENU, S)CROLL
```

The user is now able to add another item for tracking, to delete or change an existing item, return to the MENU, or scroll to subsequent projects, if more than one screen's worth are on file. Our choice in the present example will be to return to the MENU. This is accomplished by typing "M" and pressing the RETURN key. The following PRINTING OPTIONS SCREEN appears:

```
PRINTING OPTIONS

PLEASE CHOOSE ONE OF THE FOLLOWING:

1.   LISTING BY NUMBER
2.   LISTING BY STARTING DATE
3.   LISTING BY TARGET DATE
4.   LISTING BY LEAD

5.   RETURN TO MAIN MENU

?
```

The user initiates printing by typing "1" and pressing the RETURN key. This will yield the following screen:

```
PRINT HEADINGS
--------------

1.   GENERAL HOSPITAL
2.   PROJECT TRACKING SYSTEM
3.   STAN SCHMENGE
4.   ASSISTANT ADMINISTRATOR
5.   MAY 12, 1983

WOULD YOU LIKE TO    1) ALTER A HEADING?
               OR    2) PRINT AS IS?
```

The user can elect to alter the existing print heading line by line or print the report using the existing heading. If the latter is chosen, the user types "2" and presses the RETURN key. If the user desires to change the existing heading or create a new heading, if none exists, the user types "1" and presses the RETURN key. In our example we'll select the latter choice in order to demonstrate how to create or change a print heading.

The following message appears at the bottom of the screen described in the last display:

```
ENTER THE HEADING NUMBER TO BE ALTERED
```

The user can enter any line number (for up to five lines of text). This moves the cursor to that line number. If a new heading is being created, the user would start with line "1" and proceed through as many lines as are necessary to create the heading. If a change is being made to an existing heading, the appropriate line number(s) are selected one at a time and the changes made. Once the user is satisfied with the print heading, the user selects the PRINT AS IS choice, number "2." The following message appears:

```
DO YOU WANT TO INCLUDE THE NOTES?
```

If the user does not want to print the notes related to each item, the word "NO" is typed. If the notes are desired, "YES" is typed. Exhibit 6-2 shows the project list without notes and Exhibit 6-3 shows the same projects with notes. In both cases, the projects are listed in numerical

---

Exhibit 6-2 Project Tracking: Project List

GENERAL HOSPITAL
PROJECT TRACKING SYSTEM
STAN SCHMENGE
ASSISTANT ADMINISTRATOR
MAY 12

PROJECT TITLE	START	TARGET	RANK	CONTACT/LEAD
MOVE DINING ROOM EQUIPMENT	02/23/83	02/28/83	1	W. WALL
INSTALL NEW DISCHARGE PLANNING SYS	02/25/83	8/1/83	1	S.SCHMANGE
CREATE POSTER FOR MARKETING	03-01-83	3-10-83	1	J. MIRO
CHANGE ALL LIGHTING -3W	03-03-83	06-30-83	2	A.G.BELL
IMPLEMENT SALARY PROGRAM.	03-10-83	06-30-83	1	F. MAMMON
PROCURE FLOOR MATS	10/01/82	04/01/83	2	T. BOIL
CLEAN SCREENS	05/03/83	06/01/83	2	FISHER

Exhibit 6-3 Project Tracking: Project List with Notes

GENERAL HOSPITAL
PROJECT TRACKING SYSTEM
STAN SCHMENGE
ASSISTANT ADMINISTRATOR
MAY 12

PROJECT TITLE	START	TARGET	RANK	CONTACT/LEAD
MOVE DINING ROOM EQUIPMENT	02/23/83	02/28/83	1	W. WALL
	TRUCKING COMPANY CONTACTED 2/25/83			
INSTALL NEW DISCHARGE PLANNING SYS	02/25/83	8/1/83	1	S.SCHMANGE
	ORDER CABBAGE ROLLS 2-28-83 ORDER COFFEE 2-28-83 ORDERED POLKA BAND 2-28-83			
CREATE POSTER FOR MARKETING	03-01-83	3-10-83	1	J. MIRO
	ADVERTISING FIRM HIRED 3-3-83			
CHANGE ALL LIGHTING -3W	03-03-83	06-30-83	2	A.G.BELL
	DESIGN STAFF CONTACTED -3-8-83 DESIGN COMPLETED 3-26-83 CONTRACTOR HIRED 4-5-83			
IMPLEMENT SALARY PROGRAM.	03-10-83	06-30-83	1	F. MAMMUN
	DETERMINE AVERAGE PERCENT INCREASE			
PROCURE FLOOR MATS	10/01/82	04/01/83	2	T. BOIL
	CONTACT HOUSEKEEPING (10/1) DETERMINE NEEDS CONTACT PURCHASING/GET VENDORS WRITE PO/GET BIDS ACCEPT VENDOR ARRANGE FOR INSTALLATION			
CLEAN SCREENS	05/03/83	06/01/83	2	FISHER
	CONTACT HOUSEKEEPING (5/5) DETERMINE NEEDS (5/10) WRITE PO (5/11) ACCEPT BIDS/CHOOSE VEND (5/25) ARRANGE FOR CLEANING (5/25)			

order. The user should remember to set the printer before pressing the RETURN key to start printing. When the list has been printed, the program returns the user to the MENU screen.

The systems described above are examples of the many tracking functions that can be supported by microcomputers in a health care setting. Hospital administrators and managers can and should take advantage of these economically produced capabilities.

There are several canned software systems on the market that can be used effectively for project tracking. While they may require more time to learn than the spreadsheet programs, they are nevertheless very useful in situations not requiring the development of tailor-made systems. The drawbacks to these systems consist mainly of the need for users to accept their internal operating conventions. For example, the labels available to the user for various functions might be limited to those provided by the system. In addition the sort routines are usually fixed; the user must accept them. However, even with the constraints these systems might contain (such constraints are usually required in the development of general purpose software), the economy and time savings from buying such a system rather than designing your own is probably significant. Programs such as VisiSchedule and Data Factory are worth close examination.

Regardless of the manner in which they are handled, project tracking and scheduling systems are without doubt some of the more beneficial programs that can be supported by microcomputers.

FACILITIES MANAGEMENT: FACILITIES SPACE INVENTORY

Microcomputers are ideally suited for many limited data base management tasks. One is that of a facility manager, keeping track of statistics and data relating to the physical space of a hospital.

As we have seen, spreadsheet programs can be used to provide a limited data base management tool for this purpose. However, it would be better to provide several additional functions: more data per record and the capability of sorting information readily. Canned data base management programs are capable of handling this task; however, if possible, it is preferable to develop a program that will provide this function in a way suited to the particular facility.

The Facilities Space Inventory is such a program. Developed by the authors and written in the Pascal language, the program provides support both at a terminal and in printed output. The system requirements are as follows:

Hardware
Apple II 64K Microcomputer and Monitor
80 column card (Pascal compatible)
2 disk drives
Printer
Software
Apple Pascal

Upon booting the program, the first screen introduces the program, giving the version number, date of revision, and copyright information. Pressing the return key brings the user to the MAIN MENU of the Facilities Space Inventory:

```
FACILITIES SPACE INVENTORY
MAIN MENU



Please choose one of the following:

        1. Begin New Area
        2. Add Data to an Existing Area
        3. View/Alter Existing Data
        4. Sort Existing Data
        5. Print Reports
        6. System Maintenance
        7. Exit Program


                ?
```

The first option, that of starting a new unit, allows the user to initiate a file for the spaces relating to a particular area of the hospital. Each unit can contain up to 120 individual records (one for each space). In starting the file, the user is prompted to provide the program with a disk formatted in Pascal to keep the data on and a name for the data file. The program then initiates the storage of room records on the disk; the user is warned that this function will dominate the diskette file space. This information is provided to the user prior to file creation to ensure that even novices can use the program with little prior training; it is typical of the extensive use of comments made to the user in the program (see Exhibit 6-4).

Having started a file, the user may begin adding rooms to the file, entering information as prompted by the program. The data are gathered in regard to the following areas:

ADMINISTRATIVE RESPONSIBILITIES

Director:

Administrator:

Manager:

Building:

Unit:

ROOM NUMBER AND TYPE

Room Number:

Type-general:

Type-specific:

Number of Workstations:

Number of Square Feet:

USER INFORMATION

Major User:

Rent:

Cost per square foot:

Annual Cost of the space:

Annual revenue (if rented):

ROOM DESCRIPTION

Room information - 3 lines:

HOUSEKEEPING

Housekeeping Supervisor for Unit:

Room Class (housekeeping):

Position Number of Custodian responsible:

```
Time of Cleaning:

Time Trash is emptied:

Floor covering (eg., carpet):


FACILITIES/MAINTENANCE

Maintenance Supervisor:

Number of Water Outlets:

Number of Electrical Outlets:

Number of Telephone Outlets:

Space provided with sprinklers (Y/N):

Fixed Equipment:


SECURITY ARRANGEMENTS

Security Officer (Supervisor):

Time the Room is Opened:

Time the Room is Closed:

Access provided to:

Movable Equipment: (2 lines)
```

Exhibit 6-4 Facilities Space Inventory: New File

```
FACILITIES SPACE INVENTORY
INITIATE A FILE FOR A NEW AREA


** WARNING! **
This area of the program creates a disk file capable of
storing data for up to 120 rooms.  The diskette used should
be properly formatted for Pascal, and must be entirely blank
to allow for file storage.


To continue, press <return>
To return to main menu, type "q" for quit, then <return>
```

These data are entered into the program through the use of a special input screen, shown in Exhibit 6-5. This screen is used throughout the program for both input and output of space information.

The program is written to be used both as a keeper of the data base (with the associated reports) and as a dynamic source of information about the physical space of a hospital. Exhibit 6-6 shows the printed report based on the data base; it reproduces the screen, two rooms to a page. Using the sort option, data on rooms can be printed by particular characteristics.

In addition, selected fields can be printed from a given record, along with the associated room numbers. If a manager wanted a list of all current regulatory agency citations for his or her facility to add to a management report, it would be an easy matter to sort, collate, and print out such information. Additional uses can be developed for this function. The citation report is shown in Exhibit 6-7. A summary type report can be printed, showing the room number, room type, and square footage (see Exhibit 6-8).

This same feature can be used on a dynamic basis to find rooms within a facility with particular characteristics. For example, suppose a new program has been proposed requiring that a space in each area be made available for a certain function; let's say, a satellite pharmacy. The program could be used to scan the data base for rooms with the necessary characteristics (water outlet, telephone conduit, sprinkler system, minimum square footage). The additional data regarding fixed equipment and floor cover would indicate sources of additional expense in modifying the room and the data on cost could provide an estimate of lost "revenue" due to rent (typically stated as a contra-expense).

The printed version of the report (sorted by user) can be used to keep the occupants of the spaces informed about the services available. This feature is also helpful in the ongoing process of reviewing information to ensure that all spaces and services are accurately reflected in the data base.

Administrators and managers can use the Facilities Space Inventory as a quick reference to the characteristics of all spaces. The printed report can be made available on a quarterly or semiannual basis to personnel without computers in their immediate area; the program diskette and its associated data diskettes can be given to staff members with microcomputer support.

ENVIRONMENTAL QUALITY ASSURANCE PROGRAM

Environmental quality assurance is another area in which microcomputers can contribute a great deal. Although there is no easy solution to

Exhibit 6-5 Facilities Space Inventory: Data Entry Screen

```
Last change:              Facilities Space Inventory     Revised:

Director::                  Room Number:            Major User:
Admin.:                     Type-Gen.:              Rent:
Manager:                    Type-Spec:              Cost:
Building:                   Workstations:           Ann. Cost:
Unit:                       Square feet:            Ann. Income:

Room Description: ...............................................................
 ..........................................................................
 ..........................................................................

Housekeeping:               Facilities:             Security:
Room Class:                 Water:                  Room Open:
Custodian:                  Telephone:              Room Close:
Cleaned:                    Electrical:             Access:
Trash:                      Sprinkled:              Movable..:
Floor Cover:                Fixed Equip:            ..Equip:

Regulatory Agency Citations:.................................................
 ..........................................................................
 ..........................................................................

Press Return to continue...
```

Exhibit 6-6 Facilities Management: Space Inventory Report

```
Last change:05/01/83   Facilities Space Inventory     Revised:05/01/83

Director:Alpha              Room Number:3201        Major User:Hospital
Admin.: Beta                Type-Gen.:Patient       Rent:None
Manager:Gamma               Type-Spec:Semi-p        Cost:10.00
Building:Hospital           Workstations:2          Ann. Cost:1750.00
Unit:3 West                 Square feet:175         Ann. Income:0

Room Description: Typical semi-private room.  Renovated 1975, TV
installed on west wall.

Housekeeping:Smith          Facilities:Jones        Security:Cassidy
Room Class:Patient          Water:1                 Room Open:A
Custodian:08                Telephone:1             Room Close:N
Cleaned:10:00am             Electrical:6            Access:Staff, Pt.
Trash:2:00pm                Sprinkled:N             Movable..:Bed, stand
Floor Cover:Carpet          Fixed Equip:N           ..Equip:

Regulatory Agency Citations: None at this time.
```

```
Last change:05/01/83   Facilities Space Inventory   Revised:05/01/83

Director:Alpha            Room Number:3203       Major User:Staff
Admin.:Beta               Type-Gen.:Storage      Rent:0
Manager:Gamma             Type-Spec:Clean        Cost:10.00
Building:Hospital         Workstations:0         Ann. Cost:1250.00
Unit:3 West               Square feet:125        Ann. Income:0

Room Description:Supplies stored in this space include Medical/Surgical,
Pharmacy, and general items for patient care.  The crash cart for the
unit is also in this space.

Housekeeping:Smith        Facilities:Jones       Security:Cassidy
Room Class:Utility        Water:0                Room Open:A
Custodian:08              Telephone:0            Room Close:N
Cleaned:2:00pm            Electrical:2           Access:Staff
Trash:1:00pm,7:00pm       Sprinkled:N            Movable..:Arrest Cart
Floor Cover:Tile          Fixed Equip:Shelves    ..Equip:Exch. Cart

Regulatory Agency Citations:Have sign installed outside room indicating
Arrest Cart.  Install sprinkler system.  Both covered on Construction
Work Order #23432 written 04/01/83.
```

Exhibit 6-7 Facilities Management: Citations Program

```
Regulatory Agency Citations  --  Level 3
                                 05/01/83

Rm* 3201  None
Rm* 3202  None
Rm* 3203  Have sign installed outside room
          indicating Arrest Cart. Install sprinkler
          system. Both covered on Construction
          Work Order *23432 written 04/01/83
Rm* 3204  None
Rm* 3205  None
Rm* 3206  None
Rm* 3207  None
Rm* 3208  None
Rm* 3209  None
Rm* 3210  None
Rm* 3211  None
```

this complex issue, micros can do much at the local level to help improve the safety and appearance of the hospital environment. The program described was developed by the authors and run on an inexpensive Apple II-based system.

The first step in setting up an environmental quality assurance program is to identify certain general areas in which a standard of quality might be defined; a typical approach would be to divide them up by service area, as follows: Housekeeping, Maintenance, Environmental Health and Safety, and Security.

The next step would be to break down each area into the individual services provided by each service department and then develop some quantitative measure regarding the degree to which the service has been performed. For example, if Housekeeping is to dust the tops of the bedside tables daily, and keep them free of dust, a quantitative measure might be imposed on the level of performance as follows:

0—Unacceptable, service not provided
5—Some effort has been made, service still not provided
10—Acceptable, service has been provided satisfactorily

Exhibit 6-8 Facilities Management: Unit Summary Report

Facilities Space Inventory
Unit Summary for 6 West
Run Date: 08/17/83

Room Number	Manager	Room Type	Square Feet	Major User	Work Stations
W6501	Christensen	Patient - Semi	210	Dermatology	2
W6502	Christensen	Patient - Semi	210	Dermatology	2
W6503J	Christensen	Custodian	35	Housekeeping	1
W6504	Christensen	Patient - Semi	210	Dermatology	2
W6505	Christensen	Patient - Semi	210	Dermatology	2
W6506	Christensen	Nurse Station	187	Nursing	8
W6507	Christensen	Medication	67	Nursing	3
W6508	Christensen	Clean Storage	110	Nursing	0

This particular measure has been chosen because it is simple and tends to help avoid value judgments regarding the degree to which service departments meet their obligations.

Once a service standard of performance has been chosen, the standard is then applied to all of the services to be provided in a space by the department; in Housekeeping the full list of things cleaned may be as follows (not all services are performed in every room): floor cover, walls, baseboard, window sill, window tracks, window blinds, horizontal surfaces, ashtrays, doors, high dusting, phone, vents, waste receptacles, trash pulled, linen pulled, linen hamper, furnishings, sink, mirror, urinal, toilet, paper supply, fixtures, tub, shower, drinking fountain, fire cabinet, bed, bedside stand, overbed table, IV poles.

The particular items provided by the other services are more difficult to define precisely; in the program used failure to provide the service is noted through a special comment feature that allows these difficulties to be collated for all rooms in an area by service department.

The final aspect of the program to be decided upon is the frequency of inspections. Given the fact that the detailed examination can be time consuming, the inspections are done only once per month (or less, depending on the availability of personnel to perform inspections).

When the program is run, an introductory screen appears, naming the program and providing the version number and date of the program along with relevant copyright information. Upon pressing RETURN, the MAIN MENU appears, as follows:

```
ENVIRONMENTAL QUALITY ASSURANCE PROGRAM
MAIN MENU



Please choose one of the following:

      A. Define a new unit
      B. View/Alter existing unit information

      C. Enter inspection data
      D. View/Alter existing inspection data

      E. Printed reports
      F. Exit this program


                        > ? <
```

When running the program for the first time, the user must define a new unit. A unit consists of a group of rooms that will form a "set" for inspection reporting purposes.

The user is prompted to supply a properly formatted Pascal diskette and a filename for the unit. Having entered an appropriate filename, the user should enter all of the rooms necessary; the following data must be entered for each room:

```
Room Number:

Housekeeping Room Class:

Square Feet:

Floor Cover:

Cleaning time:

Supervisor:

Custodian (Position Control Number):
```

Having entered this basic information about the physical aspects of the space and those responsible for providing housekeeping service, the user must choose from the list of inspection criteria defined above (i.e., floor cover, walls, etc.) the services that will be performed in a given room. All of the services are listed on the screen, and the cursor jumps from one item to another as the user types "y" to indicate that this service is expected or "n" if not.

After this data is entered, the program will send the data to the file located on the appropriate diskette; the user will then be prompted to either add more data or to quit if done.

The second menu choice (View/Alter existing unit information) allows the user to check on the data provided for each section and change it as necessary as the purpose of the space changes over time.

The user may choose at this time to skip to menu choice E and select the appropriate item to print out a full room-by-room inspection form with blanks to allow the inspector to fill in the rating given to each service in each room.

The next set of choices allows the user to enter inspection reports for a given area. The user is prompted for a disk name and a filename, as usual, as well as the date of the inspection and the name of the person performing the inspection. As the user moves through the list of rooms, the screen changes to reflect the data entered for each area; the screen in Exhibit 6-9 illustrates the manner in which inspection data are entered.

The user would start with the cursor placed next to floor cover and check the inspection form to see the 0, 1, or 2 rating given that service for that room. The cursor then moves to the next service that is marked with a "y"—in this case, wall washing. The cursor moves in this way throughout the screen, avoiding the areas marked "n," indicating that this service is not provided in the room.

Following the entry of the housekeeping data, the user is prompted by an additional screen to type in data relating to the other service areas. For example, if a ceiling tile was missing in the room inspected, the following note would be typed into the machine:

M Loose ceiling tile in SE corner

The "M" prefix will allow the computer to separate all maintenance items from any other comments that might have been entered during this inspection period. Suitable prefixes can be assigned to comments made regarding security, environmental health, and even matters requiring special housekeeping attention.

After the inspection data have been entered, the user may choose the printed report section of the program and have a room-by-room printout of the inspection data entered, complete with a summary for that room (see Exhibit 6-10). This summary shows the full data base entered, as well as totals, average score, and percentage of acceptability (summary score divided by total possible score, times 100 percent).

Also available is a summary by unit; this report gives the same summary results as the single room report but gives the average score on each criterion rather than a particular room score (Exhibit 6-11).

In addition, it is possible to prepare a report similar to the unit summary report for each custodian. Because each of the inspection reports contains a position control number for the custodian who is primarily responsible for the appearance of the space, the inspection reports can be sorted based on each number, allowing an overview of each employee's performance.

The final report printed goes through the "comments" file and pulls out all of the remarks regarding maintenance, security, and environmental health, and prints them out, by category, with the associated room number.

In summary, the Environmental Quality Assurance Program provides the user with the following tools in the constant effort to maintain standards in a facility:

Exhibit 6-9 Environmental Quality Assurance: Inspection Data

```
ENVIRONMENTAL QUALITY ASSURANCE PROGRAM

Room Number:

Floor cover:y        Walls:y              Baseboard:y          Window Sill:y
Window track:y       Window Blinds:y      Horiz. surface:y     Ashtray:n
Door:y               High Dust:y          Phone:y              Waste Recep:y
Trash Pulled:y       Linen Pulled:n       Linen Hamper:n       Furnishing:y
Sink:y               Mirror:y             Urinal:n             Toilet:y
Paper Supply:y       Fixtures:y           Tub:n                Shower:n
Fountain:n           Fire Cabinet:n       Bed:y                Bedside Stand:y
Overbed Table:y      IV Poles:y

Please enter inspection data for this room.  The program will skip
those criteria not rated.
```

Exhibit 6-10 Environmental Quality Assurance: Room Inspection Summary

```
                    GENERAL HOSPITAL
        ENVIRONMENTAL QUALITY ASSURANCE PROGRAM

Unit: 3 East
Room Number: 3405
Inspected by: Christensen

Run Date: 05/01/83               Supervisor: Smith
Inspection Date: 04/28/83       Custodian: 08

Room Class: Patient
Square Feet: 192
Floor Cover: Carpet

Housekeeping
------------

Floor cover: 5           Walls: 10               Baseboard: 10
Window sill: 0           Window Tracks: 0       Window Blinds: 0
Surfaces: 5              Ashtrays: N            Doors: 5
High Dust: 10             Phone: 10               Vents: 5
Waste Recep.: 10          Trash: 0               Linen Recep.: N
Linen: N                 Furnishings: 5         Sink: 10
Mirror: 10                Urinal: N              Toilet: 5
Paper: 5                 Fixtures: 5            Tub: N
Shower: N                Fountain: 5            Fire Cabinet: N
Bed: 5                   Bedside st.: 10         Overbed table: 10
IV Pole: N
```

```
Items Checked: 22        Summary Score: 135        Highest Possible:
220

            #     %

zeroes:     4    18
fives:      9    41                 Average:
tens:       9    41                 Percent: 60


Housekeeping:

Maintenance:

Security:

Environmental Health:
```

Exhibit 6-11 Environmental Quality Assurance: Unit Inspection Summary

```
Unit: 3 East
Summary Report

Inspected by: Christensen

Run Date: 05/01/83                Supervisor: Smith
Inspection Date: 04/28/83        Custodian: 08, 05, 04


Housekeeping
------------

Floor cover:             Walls:                  Baseboard:
Window sill:             Window Tracks:          Window Blinds:
Surfaces:                Ashtrays:               Doors:
High Dust:               Phone:                  Vents:
Waste Recep.:            Trash:                  Linen Recep.:
Linen:                   Furnishings:            Sink:
Mirror:                  Urinal:                 Toilet:
Paper:                   Fixtures:               Tub:
Shower:                  Fountain:               Fire Cabinet:
Bed:                     Bedside st.:            Overbed table:
IV Pole:
```

```
Items Checked:          Summary Score:          Highest Possible:

          #     %

zeroes:
fives:                          Average:
tens:                           Percent:


Housekeeping:

Maintenance:

Security:

Environmental Health:
```

- a quantitative method of evaluating Housekeeping performance, at the department, supervisory, and individual custodian levels
- an organized listing of facility related tasks to be performed for all departments
- a documented history of service department performance
- a single microcomputer program that prepares all paperwork associated with these management tools

FINANCIAL MANAGEMENT

As we have seen, canned software programs can provide acceptable solutions to the problems raised while engaged in budgeting or forecasting. However, if a greater degree of user friendliness is desired, or a more precise formatting of output is needed, a custom program can provide an excellent solution.

The following program demonstrates some of the possibilities in writing one's own program. Written in 1979, and updated frequently according to changes in accounting cost centers, the program provides the following information, in three major sections:

Monthly Expenses

- Expense class—expense classes, as used by Central Accounting, for the expenditures of each account. Note that the total for commodities includes only the expenses for general and office, medical/surgical, pharmacy, and linen supplies. Because this group is more closely related to patient care (and therefore to patient days) than the other commodity items, it is advantageous to consider them as a group.
- Monthly Expense—monthly expenses for each expense class as shown by Accounting. This column does not reflect any adjustments made after the monthly deadline for submission of transfers, etc.
- Monthly Budget—amounts budgeted for each expense class for a given month according to the original annual budget sheets.
- %Var—variance (in percent) between the monthly budget and the monthly expense. When the monthly expense is greater than the monthly budget, the variance is preceded by a plus sign; when the monthly expense is less than the monthly budget, the variance is preceded by a negative sign.
- 1/12 Tot Budget—amounts that are one-twelfth of the annual budget for each expense class; that is, they indicate the "straight line" budget for that expense class.

- %Var—variance (in percent) between the "straight line" budget and the monthly expense.
- Bgt by Act Pt Days—Budget by Actual Patient Days. Amounts in this column are obtained by multiplying the amount budgeted per patient day for each expense class by the actual patient days for that month. For example, if the annual budget for medical/surgical supplies is $12,000 and the total patient days budgeted annually is 6,000, the amount budgeted for that expense class per patient day is $2.00. If the number of patient days for a given month is 500, the budget by actual patient days would be $2.00/patient day times 500 patient days, or $1,000 for that month.
- %Var—variance (in percent) between the budget by patient days and the monthly expense.

Year to Date Expenses

- Expense class—as above.
- Yr to Date Expense—expense incurred for each expense class for the year through the month of the report. The amounts are calculated directly from the monthly expenses entered each month from the budget summary received from Accounting and reflect adjustments made by the monthly deadline.
- Yr to Date Budget—amounts budgeted for each expense class for the year through the month of the report. The amounts are calculated from the monthly budget figures supplied in the budget sheets provided by Accounting.
- %Var—variance (in percent) between the year to date expense and the year-to-date budget for each expense class.
- X/12 Tot Budget—year-to-date "straight line" budget for each expense class through the month of the report. In the actual reports, the variable "X" is replaced by the number of the month; that is, the amounts shown in October (the 4th month of the fiscal year) are 4/12ths of the annual budget for each expense class.
- %Var—variance (in percent) between the year-to-date "straight line" budget and the actual year-to-date expense.
- Bgt by YTD Pt Days—amounts shown in this column are obtained by multiplying the amount budgeted per patient day for each expense class by the actual year-to-date patient days for that account.
- %Var—variance (in percent) between the total budget by patient days and the year-to-date expense.

Patient Days

- Month—months of the year, starting at the beginning of the fiscal year.

- Actual Patient Days—figures given for patient days for the unit as recorded by Admitting.
- Budgeted Pt Days—number of patient days that are projected for each month.
- %Var—variance (in percent) between the budgeted patient days and the actual patient days for each month.
- YTD Act Pt Days—year-to-date actual patient days for the unit through each month.
- YTD Bgt Pt Days—year-to-date budgeted patient days for the unit through each month.
- %Var—variance (in percent) between the year-to-date budgeted patient days and the year-to-date actual patient days for each month.
- %Tot Pt Days—percentage of the annual budgeted patient days recorded in each month.
- YTD % Pt Days—percentage of the annual budgeted patient days recorded year-to-date through the month of the report.

The resulting report is shown in Exhibit 6-12.

Running the Program

When the program is run, the following menu appears:

```
UNIT MANAGEMENT
MONTHLY VARIANCE REPORT


PLEASE CHOOSE ONE OF THE FOLLOWING:


        1. ADD NEW ACCOUNT
        2. ENTER DATA FOR EXISTING ACCOUNT
        3. ALTER EXISTING DATA
        4. PRINT VARIANCE REPORT
        5. EXIT THIS PROGRAM



                 ?
```

At this point in the first running of the program, the user should choose "1" to start a new account, or cost center, under which to enter data. The user will be prompted to supply the number of the account, which the computer will store on the diskette. The user will then be prompted to enter monthly expense budget figures as well as the annual account total

Exhibit 6-12 Financial Management: Variance Report

HOSPITAL ADMINISTRATION
APRIL VARIANCE REPORT FOR ACCOUNT 123456

EXPENSE CLASS	MONTHLY EXPENSE	MONTHLY BUDGET	% VAR	1/12 TOT BUDGET	% VAR	BGT BY ACT PT DAYS	% VAR
PRO & ADMN	991	-338	+393	751	+31.9	647	+53.1
AFSCME	484	447	+8.2	863	-43.9	743	-34.8
OFFICE	0	0	0.0	0	0.0	0	0.0
OTHER PAY	0	53	-999	53	-999	46	-999
UNBGT PAY	0	0	0.0	0	0.0	0	0.0
POSTAGE*	1	5	-80.0	3	-66.6	3	-66.6
TEL & TEL*	42	158	-73.4	284	-85.2	244	-82.7
FOOD*	58	44	+31.8	44	+31.8	38	+52.6
GEN & OFF	648	517	+25.3	637	+1.7	549	+18.0
MED/SURG	480	1089	-55.9	839	-42.7	723	-33.6
PHARMACY	541	118	+358	252	+114	217	+149
LINEN	1664	2290	-27.3	1088	+52.9	937	+77.5
UNBGT COM*	0	0	0.0	0	0.0	0	0.0
TOTAL PAY	1475	162	+810	1667	-11.5	1436	+2.7
TOTAL COM	3333	4014	-16.9	2816	+18.3	2426	+37.3

EXPENSE CLASS	YR TO DATE EXPENSE	YR TO DATE BUDGET	% VAR	10/12 TOT BUDGET	% VAR	BGT BY YTD PT DAYS	% VAR
PRO & ADMN	7996	7408	+7.9	7510	+6.4	7181	+11.3
AFSCME	4907	9190	-46.6	8630	-43.1	8251	-40.5
OFFICE	0	0	0.0	0	0.0	0	0.0
OTHER PAY	0	535	-999	530	-999	510	-999
UNBGT PAY	0	0	0.0	0	0.0	0	0.0
POSTAGE*	30	37	-18.9	30	+0.0	36	-16.6
TEL & TEL*	2258	3092	-26.9	2840	-20.4	2715	-16.8
FOOD*	268	422	-36.4	440	-39.0	427	-37.2
GEN & OFF	7589	6198	+22.4	6370	+19.1	6093	+24.5
MED/SURG	7669	7997	-4.1	8390	-8.5	8024	-4.4
PHARMACY	4366	2333	+87.1	2520	+73.2	2412	+81.0
LINEN	20961	10886	+92.5	10880	+92.6	10406	+101
UNBGT COM*	0	0	0.0	0	0.0	0	0.0
TOTAL PAY	12903	17133	-24.6	16670	-22.5	15943	-19.0
TOTAL COM	40586	27414	+48.0	28160	+44.1	26936	+50.6

* STARRED EXPENSE CLASSES NOT INCLUDED IN COMMODITY TOTALS

MONTH	ACTUAL PT DAYS	BUDGETED PT DAYS	% VAR	YTD ACT PT DAYS	YTD BGT PT DAYS	% VAR	%TOT PT DAYS	YTD % PT DAYS
JULY	617	572	+7.8	617	572	+7.8	8.8	8.8
AUGUST	621	692	-10.2	1238	1264	-2.0	8.9	17.8
SEPTEMBER	660	586	+12.6	1898	1850	+2.5	9.4	27.3
OCTOBER	690	524	+31.6	2588	2374	+9.0	9.9	37.2
NOVEMBER	527	623	-15.4	3115	2997	+3.9	7.5	44.8
DECEMBER	422	318	+32.7	3537	3315	+6.6	6.0	50.8
JANUARY	512	596	-14.0	4049	3911	+3.5	7.3	58.2
FEBRUARY	452	603	-25.0	4501	4514	-0.2	6.5	64.7
MARCH	537	601	-10.6	5038	5115	-1.5	7.7	72.4
APRIL	499	675	-26.0	5537	5790	-4.3	7.1	79.6
MAY								
JUNE								

for each of the defined expense classes. The user will then be asked to enter monthly and annual patient day budget figures.

When the entry of the annual figures for expense and patient days has been completed, the program returns the user to the MAIN MENU. The choice of menu item 2 will allow the entry of monthly actual expense figures. In this section of the program, the user is asked to choose an account from the list of started accounts and then the month of the data to be entered. The user then enters data as prompted for each expense class and then finally the actual patient-day figure for that account (or unit area).

Once again, the patient-day indicator is hard coded, but this indicator can also be easily changed in the program to whatever activity indicator is used in the department to which you wish to apply the program.

Menu item 3 gives the user the option of viewing and modifying the existing data related to budgeted expense, budgeted patient days, actual expense, and actual patient days.

Note by controlling the information entered under the initial program statements, special budgets adjusted for late transfers, corrections, etc., can be created. This will allow comparison of actual expense with budgeted expense in a more accurate and timely manner. Exhibit 6-13 presents such a sheet. The program will keep separate track of this budget with its own data file.

Menu item 4 allows the user to print the reports shown in Exhibits 6-12 and 6-13. Upon entering this area of the program, the user is prompted to choose an account number and the month for which a variance report is to be prepared. When these choices have been registered, the computer goes to the disk, obtains all of the relevant data from each month, and calculates all of the numerical entries. The completed numbers are then transferred into text strings that are then sent to the printer.

Because this program is written in BASIC, an interpreted (and therefore slow) language, it takes about three minutes to prepare the finished report. The advantage of this laborious production process is that the program can be used with virtually any printer with no modification.

In the year in which this particular program was used, a problem had arisen with respect to the budgeting scheme used by the mainframe system in preparing budget reports. Actual expense was prepared and presented in the usual way, but monthly budget figures were based on the historical expenditures of the preceding three fiscal years. Unfortunately, because of changes in the areas reported under particular accounts over the years, and adjustments that were made, the annual budget was distributed very unevenly over the year. This uneven budget spread resulted in artificial variances in most accounts.

Exhibit 6-13 Financial Management: Variance Report—Adjusted

HOSPITAL ADMINISTRATION
APRIL VARIANCE REPORT FOR ACCOUNT 123456-ADJUSTED

EXPENSE CLASS	MONTHLY EXPENSE	MONTHLY BUDGET	% VAR	1/12 TOT BUDGET	% VAR	BGT BY ACT PT DAYS	% VAR
PRO & ADMN	1159	-338	+442	751	+54.3	647	+79.1
AFSCME	484	447	+8.2	863	-43.9	743	-34.8
OFFICE	0	0	0.0	0	0.0	0	0.0
OTHER PAY	0	53	-999	53	-999	46	-999
UNBGT PAY	0	0	0.0	0	0.0	0	0.0
POSTAGE*	1	5	-80.0	3	-66.6	3	-66.6
TEL & TEL*	42	158	-73.4	284	-85.2	244	-82.7
FOOD*	58	44	+31.8	44	+31.8	38	+52.6
GEN & OFF	648	517	+25.3	637	+1.7	549	+18.0
MED/SURG	892	1089	-18.0	839	+6.3	723	+23.3
PHARMACY	485	118	+311	252	+92.4	217	+123
LINEN	2175	2290	-5.0	1088	+99.9	937	+132
UNBGT COM*	0	0	0.0	0	0.0	0	0.0
TOTAL PAY	1643	162	+914	1667	-1.4	1436	+14.4
TOTAL COM	4200	4014	+4.6	2816	+49.1	2426	+73.1

EXPENSE CLASS	YR TO DATE EXPENSE	YR TO DATE BUDGET	% VAR	10/12 TOT BUDGET	% VAR	BGT BY YTD PT DAYS	% VAR
PRO & ADMN	8163	7408	+10.1	7510	+8.6	7181	+13.6
AFSCME	4907	9190	-46.6	8630	-43.1	8251	-40.5
OFFICE	0	0	0.0	0	0.0	0	0.0
OTHER PAY	0	535	-999	530	-999	510	-999
UNBGT PAY	0	0	0.0	0	0.0	0	0.0
POSTAGE*	30	37	-18.9	30	+0.0	36	-16.6
TEL & TEL*	2258	3092	-26.9	2840	-20.4	2715	-16.8
FOOD*	268	422	-36.4	440	-39.0	427	-37.2
GEN & OFF	7589	6198	+22.4	6370	+19.1	6093	+24.5
MED/SURG	8081	7997	+1.0	8390	-3.6	8024	+0.7
PHARMACY	4310	2333	+84.7	2520	+71.0	2412	+78.6
LINEN	21472	10886	+97.2	10880	+97.3	10406	+106
UNBGT COM*	0	0	0.0	0	0.0	0	0.0
TOTAL PAY	13071	17133	-23.7	16670	-21.5	15943	-18.0
TOTAL COM	41453	27414	+51.2	28160	+47.2	26936	+53.8

* STARRED EXPENSE CLASSES NOT INCLUDED IN COMMODITY TOTALS

MONTH	ACTUAL PT DAYS	BUDGETED PT DAYS	% VAR	YTD ACT PT DAYS	YTD BGT PT DAYS	% VAR	%TOT PT DAYS	YTD % PT DAYS
JULY	617	572	+7.8	617	572	+7.8	8.8	8.8
AUGUST	621	692	-10.2	1238	1264	-2.0	8.9	17.8
SEPTEMBER	660	586	+12.6	1898	1850	+2.5	9.4	27.3
OCTOBER	690	524	+31.6	2588	2374	+9.0	9.9	37.2
NOVEMBER	527	623	-15.4	3115	2997	+3.9	7.5	44.8
DECEMBER	422	318	+32.7	3537	3315	+6.6	6.0	50.8
JANUARY	512	596	-14.0	4049	3911	+3.5	7.3	58.2
FEBRUARY	452	603	-25.0	4501	4514	-0.2	6.5	64.7
MARCH	537	601	-10.6	5038	5115	-1.5	7.7	72.4
APRIL	499	675	-26.0	5537	5790	-4.3	7.1	79.6
MAY								
JUNE								

It was therefore necessary to enter the mainframe budget figure and compare it with a straight line budget figure to show the uneven spread of budgeted funds. The micro was able to provide this additional analysis with ease.

The patient-day adjusted budget is particularly useful in demonstrating the expense classes that vary according to fluctuation in patient days. If the patient days have been reduced by 15 percent, for example, some reduction in expense would be expected.

This particular program demonstrates both the use of microcomputers to obtain figures that are not typically available from a mainframe system and the ability of small computers to respond effectively to the problems sometimes created by the uniform approach to budgeting used on large-scale systems. The major financial and activity information needed by a unit level manager is neatly summarized in a single sheet, with the capability of comparing those portions of the budget dependent on activity with the actual expenses incurred.

MEDICAL RECORDS APPLICATIONS

The medical records department is charged with the task of analyzing, cataloging, storing, retrieving, and disseminating often large numbers of patient records. It seems clear that the advent of the totally computerized medical record will be economically unfeasible in the near future. Hospitals have been attempting to develop large-scale systems to handle medical information since the 1960s. System developers eventually reached the conclusion that achieving this took longer and cost more than anyone expected. There are several specific medical records department management tasks, however, that are quite amenable to support by a microcomputer. In this section we will describe several useful programs for supporting these functions.

Chart Deficiency Tracking

Perhaps one of the most intractable problems facing medical records practitioners is that of incomplete medical records. One of the main reasons for loss of accreditation is the failure to keep medical records up to date. The Joint Commission Accreditation of Hospitals (JCAH) considers a record to be delinquent if it has not been completed within 15 days after the patient has been discharged. The medical records department plays a crucial part in assisting the medical staff to keep up to date with medical records completion. It is the department's responsibility to keep track of incomplete records and to report to the medical staff the number of outstanding incomplete and/or delinquent records so that physician control can be exercised to obtain completion.

The completion by physicians of records of discharged patients is usually considered to be a burdensome task. In most hospitals, there are always backlogs of incomplete records. These are stored and indexed in some way so they are accessible for completion and followup patient care. Generally, the records are arranged in alphabetical or numerical order and placed in boxes or bins identified by physicians' names. There is usually an alphabetical index that is used to locate the records when needed. The arrangement and indexing of records for accessibility, as well as the movement of records from one physician's box to another's, conflict with the need to provide information (usually on a weekly or bi-weekly basis) on the location of and responsibility for incomplete records.

A significant amount of clerical time may be spent in physically counting records, recording counts, posting, adding, etc., in order to provide a complete report. A large amount of typing may be required (this may result in transcription errors). Finally, envelopes must be typed, stuffed, and mailed. In large hospitals, the whole process may take so long that the information is out of date by the time the physicians receive it. There is nothing worse for an information system manager than being criticized for sending an unwarranted "dunning" letter, and nothing more gratifying for the habitual offender than to be able to carp about being treated unfairly.

The typical situation may be described as follows:

- Step 1. After the records have been reviewed for deficiencies, a slip or card is attached to each record noting the deficiencies and the doctors responsible for correcting them.
- Step 2. Index cards are prepared (typed or handwritten) indicating the location of the records. These are usually filed in alphabetical order.
- Step 3. At set intervals a physical inventory is taken of all records filed in the incomplete medical records file. A clerk enters the date and medical record identification number of each record in every physician's box or bin on some type of inventory sheet or report. Usually, a separate page is assigned to each physician.

If, after one week has elapsed, a record is still incomplete, the clerk makes a notation of this on the inventory sheet. If the record remains incomplete after two weeks, the clerk indicates the record is delinquent. The date the record was considered to have become delinquent is recorded. Only after a record has been accounted for as complete does the clerk scratch it from the inventory and remove the index card.

In some systems, there is no way to determine whether the record has been completed or merely removed from a bin for some reason. This reduces the credibility of the entire system.

• Step 4. The clerk transfers the totals for each physician, by record status, to a finished report.

• Step 5. This report is used to prepare notices of incomplete and/or delinquent records that are mailed to the medical staff. The lists may also be divided by clinical department and sent to the appropriate leadership for followup. The list may be used for punitive purposes as well, such as the denial of admitting privileges until records are completed or as a basis for "fines" to be levied.

It may take several days or more to complete these steps. There are undoubtedly many instances where because of time constraints the job is not totally completed. If punitive measures are to be taken that are based on the information thus provided, the need for timeliness and accuracy is quite apparent. Many cases of physician and medical record staff consternation occur daily, or are avoided by the medical record department "backing off" because of lack of confidence in its information.

The usual methods of tracking incomplete records are also tedious in that they force clerks to complete an onerous and boring task in one marathon session. The absence of the "crucial" clerk on inventory day can be disastrous because the entire system can collapse.

A more appropriate approach is to stretch the task into a continuous daily inventory with the reports produced by a computer whenever desired or needed. A microcomputer-supported medical records inventory and reporting system attacks the problems of inaccuracy, untimeliness, boredom, and consternation at their source. Microcomputers streamline the task, reduce time spent, and minimize the time lag between inventory and reporting. This, in turn, may help reduce the number of incomplete records and control delinquencies in record completion.

The following analogy may be useful in describing how such a system would work. In any inventory control system there are two main elements: items (such as parts, supplies, products, documents, etc.) and quantity on hand. In this case, the item is a specific physician's incomplete medical records and the quantity is, of course, the number of incomplete records "on hand." Each physician is assigned a code that corresponds to the "part" or item number. The medical record identification numbers may be considered "serial numbers." The total number of incomplete medical records assigned to any particular physician constitutes the "stock on hand" for that "item." It is thus possible to arrange the medical records in such a way as to be able to determine at any time the current "stock on hand" for each physician.

By entering this information into a microcomputer in a dynamic manner, the inventory file is established. The file can be updated continuously as activity occurs, simply by changing status information. Updating on a daily basis may take only minutes per day, and since this activity would have to be completed whether or not supported by a computer no additional real work is involved.

The following example represents one way to enhance a hospital's medical record deficiency reporting system using a "medium-sized" microcomputer capability. The following assumptions have been made:

1. The hospital has already begun to develop a cadre of people with some microcomputer knowledge or expertise, or
2. Software exists to run the programs outlined. (No such microcomputer software appears to be presently available, although mainframe computer hardware may be available. The authors are presently developing such microcomputer software.)
3. The "psychological" status of the medical records department is such that a change of this nature in its systems would be accepted and supported by the staff.

The system described is developed using a number of "phases." It may be helpful to read Appendix B before proceeding with the development of your own medical records deficiency tracking system.

Dcsign Phase

An "existing" system has been examined and found to be lacking in a number of respects. The purpose of designing a new system is to provide more up-to-date medical record deficiency information for reporting and control.

The first step is to decide what reports and information are desired or necessary. Those shown in Exhibits 6-14, 6-15, 6-16, and 6-17 are suggested. These reports include:

- chart deficiency tracking inventory by physician
- chart deficiency tracking inventory by physician/department
- chart deficiency tracking inventory—numerical reference
- chart deficiency tracking inventory—department summary

The Numerical Reference List can be used as an aid in locating medical records and is therefore helpful to the staff. In addition to these reports, the development of a method of simplifying the production of individual

Exhibit 6-14 Chart Deficiency Tracking: Inventory by Physician

MEDICAL RECORDS DEPARTMENT
INVENTORY OF INCOMPLETE RECORDS
BY RESPONSIBLE PHYSICIAN

DATE: APRIL 30
YEAR: 1983

PHYSICIAN	SERVICE	RECORD NUMBER	PATIENT	DSCH DATE	RECORD AGE
ADAMS, CHARLES	MEDICINE	343223	JOHNSON, HAROLD	3-23-83	38
		343455	CARRUTHERS, MAUDE	3-14-83	47
		343668	DIETRICH,FLORENCE	3-28-83	33
		343602	BAKER, JAMES	2-26-83	64
		343789	THOMAS, RUTH	3-25-83	36
		343801	GORDON. HARRY	4-11-83	19
		343887	FISHER, THOMAS	4-15-83	15
BOYD, OSGOOD	MEDICINE	343765	ROBERTS, FLOYD	4-15-83	15
		343881	DOAN, CATHERINE	4-12-83	18
TROJENIC, I.A.	MEDICINE	343336	SWANSON,ALICE	2-15-83	74
		343367	CLARK, GEORGE	2-14-83	73
		343459	DENNIS, BETH	2-25-83	64
		343498	SMITH, TERRY	2-28-83	61
		343562	LOMAX, PETER	3-03-83	58
		343587	ROGERS, ROY	3-14-83	47
		343599	TERHUNE, FRANCES	3-25-83	36
		343691	BILLINGS,CLYDE	3-17-83	44
		343712	YATES, SANDRA	3-29-83	32
		343882	WALTERS, RICHARD	4-11-83	19
		343901	HERMAN, FRANK	4-09-83	21
		343953	ULRICH, DANIEL	4-06-83	24
		343999	FLEMING, NEAL	4-02-83	28

letters to delinquent physicians for those hospitals that use such letters is recommended. If the number of letters is within certain limits, a microcomputer could be quite beneficial both in terms of reduced labor and improved timeliness. An example of such a letter as produced by a microcomputer is shown in Exhibit 6-18.

The next step is to define and describe the information or data elements required by the system. The data required to produce the reports listed above are as follows:

1. Medical record identification numbers
2. Dates
   A. Patient discharged
   B. Record assigned to a particular physician

Exhibit 6-15 Chart Deficiency Tracking: Inventory by Department

MEDICAL RECORDS DEPARTMENT
INVENTORY OF INCOMPLETE RECORDS
PHYSICIAN/DEPARTMENT

DATE: APRIL 30,
YEAR: 1983

DEPARTMENT	PHYSICIAN	INCOMP RECORDS	OLDEST RECORD	DELINQ ?
MEDICINE	ADAMS, STEPHEN	32	2-24-83	YES
	BAKER, ARNOLD	7	4-18-83	NO
	BENDER, TRENT	15	3-25-83	YES
	ENNIS, JOHN	23	3-26-83	YES
	GORDON, VERNON	3	4-25-83	NO
	HOBBS, THOMAS	11	4-17-83	NO
	JONES, GENE	10	4-19-83	NO
	SIMPSON, ARTHUR	24	3-30-83	YES
	TRENT, KARL	2	4-20-83	NO
TOTAL FOR DEPT.		127		

C. Current date of most recent activity (record assigned or completed)
D. Dates of all previous activity (if historical reports are desired)

3. Current status of record
4. Previous status (if historical reports are desired)
5. Physician identification (names, addresses, code numbers, medical department/division)

The information will be entered into the system via microcomputer by clerical personnel on a daily basis as activity occurs.

Programming Phase

Thus, the purpose for designing a medical records deficiency tracking system is for control through a series of informative reports. The programming necessary to produce these reports is complicated and will not be reproduced below. However, the necessary programming and file design will be explored. The programming for a medical record deficiency tracking system includes (1) a program to enable the input and massaging of information (called the Medical Record Deficiency Application Program) and (2) programs to produce the desired output (reports) (called, quite simply,

Exhibit 6-16 Chart Deficiency Tracking: Numerical Reference List

MEDICAL RECORDS DEPARTMENT
INVENTORY OF INCOMPLETE RECORDS
NUMERICAL REFERENCE LIST

DATE: APRIL 30,

YEAR: 1983

RECORD NUMBER	LOCATION IN FILE	DATE FILED	REMARKS
343112	DR. J SMITH	4-14-83	PULLED FOR CLINIC
343115	DR. F. REDDY	4-23-83	
343167	DR. G. FRY	3-24-83	
343178	DR. A. GOMEZ	4-15-83	
343179	DR. L. DOBBS	3-28-83	
343198	DR. T. EDWARDS	4-13-83	OUT TO CORRESPONDENCE
343200	DR. E. THOMAS	4-26-83	
343223	DR. J. SMITH	3-17-83	
343335	DR. H. BAUGH	4-21-83	
343226	DR. S. CLEMENS	4-10-83	
343256	DR. L. CARROLL	4-04-83	PULLED FOR CLINIC
343267	DR. B. SKINNER	4-18-83	
343287	DR. F. CASSIDY	4-20-83	
343304	DR. B. SKINNER	3-29-83	
343339	DR. F. REDDY	2-24-83	
343347	DR. F. HARRIS	4-03-83	
343365	DR. S. ULLMAN	4-21-83	
343369	DR. B. RUSSELL	4-18-83	
343387	DR. J. ROGERS	4-20-83	
343397	DR. E. SWANSON	4-25-83	
343399	DR. K. YEAGER	4-25-83	
343403	DR. H. BAUGH	4-24-83	OUT TO CORRESPONDENCE
343450	DR. E. THOMAS	4-21-83	

Medical Record Deficiency Output Programs). The design requirements are illustrated in Figure 6-1.

Appropriate algorithms to calculate time elapsed, assign physicians and appropriate departments (to generate reports), generate letters, and accept input must be devised. The time required to prepare and run these programs has not yet been determined, but they should not be considered to be of the most difficult nature.

Perhaps more difficult is the task of determining the size of the system necessary to do this job. This would, of course, depend on the size of the hospital and its medical records deficiency problem. In the best of all worlds, the problem would be quite small because physicians would have

Exhibit 6-17 Chart Deficiency Tracking: Summary

MEDICAL RECORDS DEPARTMENT
INVENTORY OF INCOMPLETE RECORDS
SUMMARY BY DEPARTMENT

DATE: APRIL 30,
YEAR: 1983

DEPARTMENT	NUMBER OF INC REC	NUMBER OF DEL REC	NUMBER OF DRS DEL
MEDICINE	398	138	34
SURGERY	354	165	38
OB/GYN	35	11	2
PEDIATRIC	143	59	6
OTORHINO	98	23	4
UROLOGY	56	21	4
DERMATOL	211	80	19
OPHTHY	51	21	2
ORTHOPED	76	43	11
PED SURG	23	34	9
THORACIC	47	2	1
GI	87	19	3
ONCOLOGY	38	4	1
ALLERGY	12	0	0
PULMONARY	31	0	0
TOTAL	1660	620	134

completed their medical record keeping responsibilities. In fact, the goal of the system being described is to eliminate most of the problem. It would, however, be a pipe dream to think that this is the usual situation in most hospitals. What is needed is a system that, given the propensity of some physicians to delay or avoid their medical record completion duties (thereby exhibiting a general human trait), will keep things from getting totally out of control.

The size of the system required to handle the task may be calculated as follows:

1. Determine the size of each "field." That is, for each information element, determine the number of characters (alphabetic, numeric, or symbolic) required for its identification.
2. Determine the total number of characters per "record." A record is a set of data comprising one or more fields.

Exhibit 6-18 Chart Deficiency Tracking: Physician Notice

MEDICAL RECORDS DEPARTMENT
GENERAL MEMORIAL HOSPITAL
122 WEST COVINGTON

NOTICE OF INCOMPLETE/DELINQUENT
MEDICAL RECORDS

DR. I.A. TROJENIC
123 WEST COVINGTON
ANYPLACE, U.S.A. 00000

05/02/83

DEAR DR. TROJENIC:

OUR RECORDS SHOW THAT AS OF 04/30/83 THERE WERE 43 INCOMPLETE MEDICAL RECORDS IN YOUR FILE. OF THESE, 21 WERE MORE THAN 15 DAYS OLD, AND ARE THEREFORE CONSIDERED TO BE DELINQUENT.

AS YOU KNOW, THE RULES OF THE MEDICAL STAFF REQUIRE PHYSICIANS TO BE UP TO DATE IN RECORD COMPLETION AS A CONDITION OF MEDICAL STAFF MEMBERSHIP. PLEASE MAKE ARRANGEMENTS TO COMPLETE THESE RECORDS NO LATER THAN THREE DAYS OF RECEIPT OF THIS NOTICE. YOUR COOPERATION IS ESSENTIAL TO YOUR CONTINUED MEMBERSHIP IN GOOD STANDING OF THE MEDICAL STAFF.

SINCERELY YOURS,

FREDERICK L. RUTHERFORD, M.D.
CHIEF OF STAFF

Thus, a record may be characterized as including the following fields:

Medical record number	7
Characters (numeric) for discharge date	8
Characters (numeric) for activity date	8
Characters (numeric) for record status	2
Characters (numeric) for physician code no.	5
Total characters (numeric)	30

Figure 6-1 Medical Records Tracking System Design

```
        *****************************************
        *  MEDICAL RECORDS DEFICIENCY TRACKING  *
        *  PROGRAM CONFIGURATION                *
        *****************************************

               ****************************
               *  RECORD STATUS UPDATING  *
               *                          *
               *  (DATA ENTRY)            *
               ****************************

                     ****************
                     *  APPLICATION *
                     *  PROGRAMS    *
                     ****************

                   *******************
                   *  MEDICAL RECORD *
                   *  DEFICIENCY     *
                   *  DATA SET       *
                   *******************

                      *************
                      *  OUTPUT   *
                      *  PROGRAMS *
                      *************

*********************************************************************
*  INVENTORY OF * INVENTORY OF *  NUMERICAL * SUMMARY * DEFICIENCY *
*   INCOMPLETE  *  INCOMPLETE  *  REFERENCE * REPORTS *  LETTERS   *
*    RECORDS    *   RECORDS    *   LISTING  *         *            *
*   (PHYSICIAN) *   (DEPT.)    *            *         *            *
*********************************************************************
```

Another file containing the actual names and addresses of the physicians, at approximately 50 characters per record, would also have to be established. A file containing, say, 200 physician addresses would occupy 10,000 character spaces, or bytes. Another file, linking the physician codes to department identification would require approximately 6,000 spaces or bytes, at 30 characters per physician record, assuming a physician staff of about 200. The actual file of incomplete records would require variable space depending on the size of the problem. For every 100 incomplete records, 3,000 bytes or characters would be required. Thus, for 1,000 records, 30,000 bytes would be required.

The average 5¼ inch floppy diskette (assuming a disk operating system is used) contains between 100,000 and 400,000 bytes of data. This means that in a system involving 200 physicians and 2,000 incomplete records, about 69,000 bytes would be required (6,000 for physician identification, 3,000 for department identification, and 60,000 for incomplete record files). All of these records could be stored on a single diskette. A small computer with processing and storage capacity of 128,000 bytes would easily store and process such a job. A smaller computer of 64,000 bytes capacity could also do the job but with somewhat more physical handling of diskettes.

To summarize, in order to determine the size of the system the following steps can be followed:

1. Determine the size of the necessary programming algorithms to be used. This number of bytes should be added to the number of bytes determined in the example above.
2. Determine the amount of data or information in each field.
3. Determine the amount of data or information in each record by adding up the numbers of characters for each field in the record.
4. Determine or estimate the largest number of incomplete records to be processed or stored at any given time. If the number of incomplete records is greater than 3,000, it is probably wise to consider some type of hard disk storage system and at least a 128,000 byte internal processing capacity. (A five Megabyte (five million bytes) hard disk system can store as much data as about thirty-five 5¼ inch floppy diskettes.)

The actual programming requires the development of algorithms that provide for the initial "managing" or processing of data. This programming effort includes setting up the data base files that include all the desired information. Two files are needed: a file containing the indicated information elements above and a physician name and address/department identification file.

The initial application programs would allow users to enter information, on a case-by-case basis, into the computer's memory or storage. Another application program would link the physician code numbers with the name and address/department identification files. This would produce what might be called the medical records deficiency information set, since it would contain all of the information required to produce the desired reports or letters to physicians. Some of the programs could take advantage of existing algorithms that are used in other settings. Other parts of the programming would have to be written from scratch. Graphic programs that produce trended information are also available for use with the medical records deficiency tracking system.

The system outlined above automatically generates medical records deficiency reports on a periodic basis that convey information on the scope of deficiencies for individual physicians. These reports may be distributed to each physician, to departmental or service chiefs, and to other appropriate administrative staff.

Benefits for Accounts Receivable

A side benefit of this system could be a reduction in the number and dollar amount of unbilled patient accounts. In many instances patient accounts cannot be billed, or collected, without complete medical record documentation. This documentation is most often provided through the transmittal of discharge summaries or other reports that document diagnostic and treatment information. Closer tracking of deficiencies in medical records documentation should reduce the number of incomplete medical records and, in turn, the number of unbilled accounts. An improvement in this area, where improvement is greatly needed, would indeed justify the initial investment required to purchase or develop a computer-supported medical records deficiency tracking and reporting system.

Department Productivity Analysis

Productivity analysis, measurement, and control are subjects that receive much attention during times of economic depression, when markets are static and revenues are shrinking in terms of fixed dollars. The application of hospital revenue-containing strategies such as Diagnosis Related Groups is intended, as a matter of policy, to encourage price competition and improved productivity. There are, of course, many methods to describe and scrutinize productivity. Such investigations can occur at macroeconomic levels involving entire national economies, at the level of specific industries, or at the level of the firm, department, or individual production element. Here, we will concern ourselves with a particular application that can be used to support the measurement, analysis, and reporting of productivity in a medical records department setting. Such a system can be easy to develop and simple to maintain.

The system helps measure production in terms of work or effort, output, and standards. These standards may be derived historically by using existing information or through engineering studies. Quite often the establishment of productivity standards comes about as a result of negotiation between departmental management and hospital administration.

Productivity may be approached from a number of different, valid perspectives, including economics, industrial engineering operations research, behavioral science, and management science. The productivity analysis that follows adopts the industrial engineering perspective. The system to be described can have greatest utility in medium to large hospitals or health care organizations; it has applicability to organizations of any size.

The relationships of labor productivity to other measurable factors that complete the productivity measurement "equation" (such as capital or commodities) should be kept in mind. It would make little sense to believe that the simple measurement of output per hour or day tells the whole story. The application of capital may play a large part in the ultimate output of a system in relation to the impact of such applications on labor. Thus, while labor might produce one level of output before the introduction of a labor-saving device, its introduction might enhance output far beyond present capacities and at reduced total cost. While the medical records department is typically labor intensive, many capital tools such as word processing equipment, high-speed photocopy equipment, computers, and, indeed, microcomputers can be used to increase productivity as well as to improve quality.

Supply costs do not usually exceed more than 30 to 35 percent of a medical records department's operating budget. Though these costs are measurable, they may be less controllable than labor or capital costs. Moreover, the department can usually complete its assigned tasks in a variety of ways. Changes in methods can often result in positive or negative changes in production or productivity. The effects of changing external demands for medical record keeping and information reporting, most often created by the requirements of third-party reimbursement (Blue Cross, Medicare, Medicaid) or regulatory bodies (JCAH, departments of public health, health planning agencies) can be damaging to medical records department budgets as well as productivity. Tracking the effects of such changes and taking steps if possible to ameliorate their effects on productivity through changes in methods should be a goal of the well-managed department. In the same vein, the need for additional personnel may often be hidden or overlooked if standards of performance don't exist or if a department's output is not being measured. In such a case staffing may not be adjusted to meet the new demand. Of course, it is necessary to measure changes that indicate downward as well as upward trends. In either case lack of measurement forecloses on management's ability to make appropriate budget adjustments.

Running the Program

The technique presented for the medical records department is simple and easy to use in measuring and tracking productivity. It utilizes the microcomputer's capacity to manipulate and store large quantities of data rapidly, thus reducing a burdensome manual task. The process provides department management with a less "painful" procedure for tracking labor productivity in a timely and analytical way.

Many medical records departments without doubt engage in measuring productivity. This is one reason this department has been chosen as a prime example of how such measurements can be meaningful and helpful. Other reasons for using medical records as an example are that the tasks performed are usually discrete; criteria and standards of performance can be derived through analysis, and changes in methods that result from external demands or internal efforts to improve can be organized, understood, and controlled. Let us begin by outlining the steps required to measure medical records department labor productivity.

1. The tasks to be performed by the department must be identified.
2. The output to be produced must be estimated in terms of work product.
3. The labor input or effort required to produce some measurable part of the output must be analyzed and formally established.
4. Performance standards based on actual department activity must be established. Several methods can be used, including analysis of historical data if it exists, the adoption of existing standards in comparable institutions, or the engineering of standards through time and motion study or short interval analysis. The engineering approach is preferable, if resources permit, because the results are more likely to accurately reflect the department's existing situation.
5. Calculations must be made of actual production for comparative purposes. This involves multiplying the number of units produced by the standard indicator of "credit" earned per unit (the credit is shown in terms of "hours earned"); this quantity is divided by the

actual number of productive hours (or total hours worked). The answer is the percent of labor productivity.

Exhibit 6-19 illustrates a productivity analysis model for the medical records department. Activities such as telephone calls, delivery trips, or other travel by employees, preparation and setup of work, etc., are contained within each production standard in a manner that makes it possible to analyze and report the total labor input and output of the department.

Additional Benefits

By employing a spreadsheet program such as VisiCalc to perform the calculations and store results required to track productivity over time, the

---

Exhibit 6-19 Department Productivity Analysis: Task List

MEDICAL RECORDS DEPARTMENT

Period: Week of Feb. 13, 1983

TASK	ACTIVITY	STD HRS	EARNED HRS	HRS W'KED	INDEX
Records Abstracted	500	.33	165	160	101
Records Filed	1400	.02	28	32	89
Corresp.	480	.25	120	120	100
Records Tr'scribed	520	.50	260	320	80
Records Coded	500	.10	50	50	100
Records Combined	500	.10	50	50	100
Records Analyzed	500	.125	63	60	102
Totals			736	792	93

TYPICAL WEEKLY TASKS NOT USUALLY ITEMIZED ABOVE:

Court Appearances, meetings, etc. = SCHEDULED HRS = 14
HRS USED = 12

Grand Totals			750	804	
93					

Exhibit 6-20 Department Productivity Analysis: Periodic Report

MEDICAL RECORDS DEPARTMENT

PRODUCTION SUMMARY REPORT

PERIOD	EARNED HOURS	WORKED HOURS	PRODUCT INDEX	O.T. WORKED	VAC. HOURS	SICK HOURS	TOTAL HOURS	BUDGET HOURS	PERCENT BUDGET
NOV 82	2108	2213	0.95	0	32	48	2341	2380	98.36
DEC 82	2113	2001	1.06	0	246	58	2363	2380	99.29
JAN 83	2004	2100	0.95	0	134	60	2354	2380	98.91
FEB 83	2345	2299	1.02	0	0	52	2403	2380	100.97
MAR 83	2310	2245	1.03	0	0	36	2317	2380	97.35
APR 83	2296	2276	1.01	0	0	43	2362	2380	99.24
MAY 83	2341	2211	1.06	0	32	61	2365	2380	99.37
JUN 83	1990	2004	0.99	0	256	39	2338	2380	98.24
TOT YTD	17507	17349	1.01	0	700	397	18843	19040	98.97

Figure 6-2 Department Productivity Analysis: Line Graph

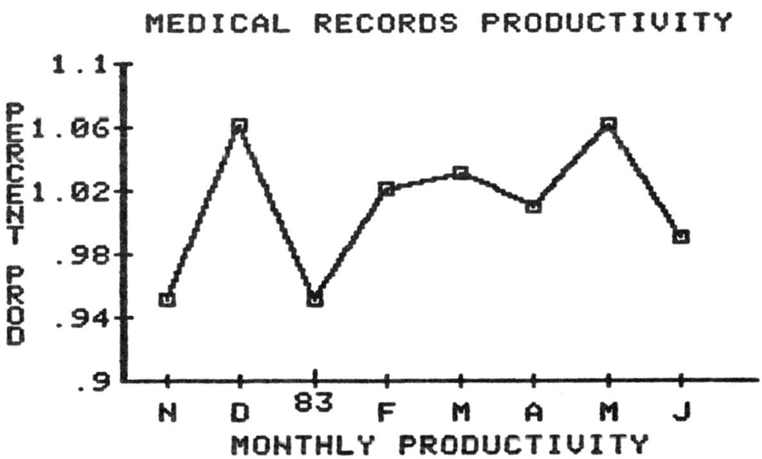

need to recalculate aggregate quantities in each column is eliminated. The work involved in performing the calculations is drastically, almost amazingly, reduced.

The data produced in the individual task productivity analysis can be used to provide periodic reports on overall department productivity (see Exhibit 6-20). The same information may be presented graphically as shown in Figure 6-2.

Awareness is the key to good management. With this program the department head and administrator will be able to analyze and control staffing through accurate and timely tracking of changes in the volume of output and work related to productivity.

The program described above is simple to develop, using the instructions provided in Chapter 4. In addition to the spreadsheet package, the system requires a 64K microcomputer with a reasonably fast printer (dot-matrix printers are preferred for spreadsheet production, although the slower, inexpensive letter-quality printers will do quite nicely). The spreadsheet approach is simpler than the dynamic programming approach in that the software exists and can be purchased at reasonable cost. A tailored program may be somewhat easier to use but more expensive and difficult to produce. However, the economics of any individual situation may dictate the wisdom of providing a custom programming effort in order to make the system applicable to a number of departments. This would achieve the economies required by the larger programming task.

Chapter 7

Microcomputer Graphics

The management of large quantities of data is one of the tasks at which microcomputers excel. However, the problem of assimilating all of this added information, and finding meaning therein, is not quite as simple. Many people are unable to glance at a meticulously prepared table of figures and immediately grasp the trends hidden in the numbers. The microcomputer can help with this task by using its graphics capabilities. In this chapter, we will examine the use of graphics software with micros.

HARDWARE/SOFTWARE REQUIREMENTS

The hardware requirements for graphics are somewhat different from those for text processing and electronic spreadsheets. As you may recall, in Chapter 2 we examined the screen characteristics that are desirable in a word processor. One of the most important had to do with how many characters could be placed on the screen at a time; most of the more professional systems allow the use of a screen "measuring" 80 characters wide by 24 lines long for a total of 1,920 characters per screen.

There is an equivalent sort of standard for graphics presentation on computers. The measure involves the number of pixels (or "dots") of light that can be controlled by the machine, rather than the number of characters. Actually, if you look closely, you can see that the characters on the screen are themselves made up of small dots. In a way, text processing uses a sort of specialized high resolution graphics.

Most of the micros in use can handle a graphics display of approximately 200×250 pixels or better, for a total of about 50,000 controllable points. The importance of the number of pixels lies in the resolution that they give. The more pixels per square inch on the screen, the finer the image that can be reproduced.

Depending on the computer, the capability to produce graphic images may be sold as a package or added on with a special card. Be sure to check with the dealer regarding the system purchased.

Having obtained a microcomputer capable of producing a sufficiently detailed image, the next step is to purchase the software capable of producing the graphics needed. It is possible to program micros to draw pictures yourself; however, it is a very time-consuming chore, given the excellent programs commercially available.

Some of the features provided in today's graphics packages are as follows:

- line, bar, area, pie, scatter, hi/lo graphs
- titles placed at top, sides, bottom; legends
- edit, load, save, manipulate files of data points
- save pictures to disk, or print

In addition, some of the higher-priced systems may include the following capabilities:

- movable titles placed anywhere on graphic
- regressions, statistical analysis, and transformation of data sets by user-defined equations
- utilization of files created by other programs (e.g., from spreadsheets)
- placement of two graphs side by side, or overlay graphs
- 3-D type bar graphs
- completed graphs transferable to other programs (e.g., a memo on a word processing program)

An excellent example of the software available is provided by VisiCorp's VisiPlot/VisiTrend program; most of the graphs shown in this book were prepared using this program. Upon entering the program, the user is presented with the menu of overall capabilities; one may choose to load files from a disk, create new files, or create graphs. The program also does a fine job of aiding the user in keeping track of data files.

Consider the following example. Suppose you wanted to graph the information contained in Exhibit 7-1, You would simply enter the edit portion of the program, and start a new file for each set of points, giving each a separate name (i.e., "actual" and "budget"). Typically, one must also specify the time period (i.e., weeks, months) over which the data are presented. Having defined the file, you would type in the data points.

Exhibit 7-1 Budgeted and Actual Expense: Data Points

	Budgeted Expense	Actual Expense
January	$ 23,456	$ 25,666
February	21,156	24,810
March	22,894	25,103
April	24,813	25,183
May	25,499	25,871
June	27,125	28,144
July	33,452	35,221
August	22,543	24,513
September	19,222	23,456
October	21,235	21,144
November	24,987	28,155
December	29,135	31,133

At this point, you would move to the plot portion of the program and choose the kind of graph that will appear; i.e., line, scatter, pie, or bar graph. Then the sets of data points to be graphed are selected from those in the computer's internal memory. If another set is needed from disk, that loading can take place.

Given the data points and the graph type requested, the computer does all of the work in preparing the graph. An esthetically pleasing axis size and axis divisions are all computed by the screen and then plotted for the user to view and customize as needed.

The finished graph appears in Figure 7-1. Notice that it is a simple line graphic, with only the barest quantity of titles or other information. This can be easily remedied by moving to the appropriate section of the program and adding titles and other relevant facts. The result is shown in Figure 7-2.

Figure 7-1 Budgeted and Actual Expense: Line Graph

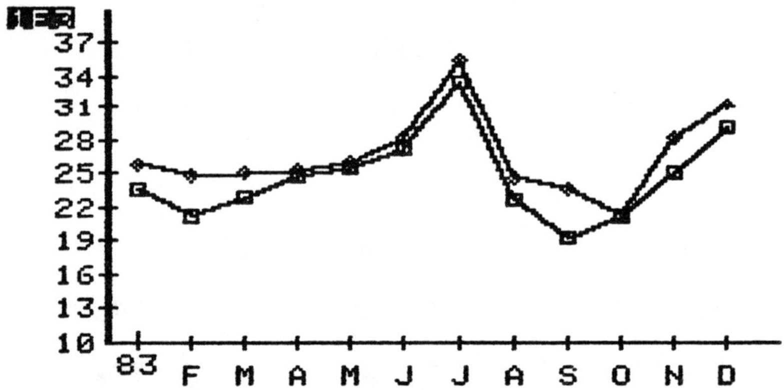

Figure 7-2 Budgeted and Actual Expense: Detailed Line Graph

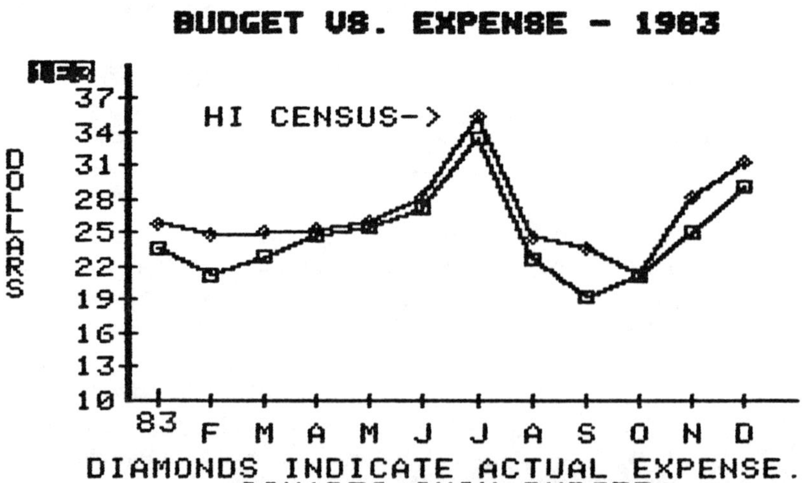

Bold and plain print, the ability to maneuver small titles to the proper points on the graph, and appropriate axis labels are all good features to look for in a graphics program. In terms of the kinds of graphs that can be done, microcomputers are still somewhat limited; however, most of the graphs that are useful in business are available.

As for manipulating the data points entered, suppose that we wanted to make obvious the cumulative effect of the unfavorable variance that is shown in this hypothetical account. This can be done by massaging the old data sets into new ones consisting of monthly year-to-date totals. The resulting data sets are shown in Figure 7-3.

Another helpful feature of a good graphics program is that it will allow you to print out a copy of the new data sets for your records, as shown in Exhibit 7-2.

Also, in purchasing a graphics program, it is a good idea to see if the program will accept sets of points from another program. For example, if you have already calculated a long series of points on a spreadsheet, it is much more convenient (and accurate) to transfer them directly to the graphics program.

ADMITTING STATISTICS

The major advantage of using a graph over a table is that it can literally provide a better picture of the information. For example, we could have

Figure 7-3 Cumulative Effect of Variance: Bar Graph

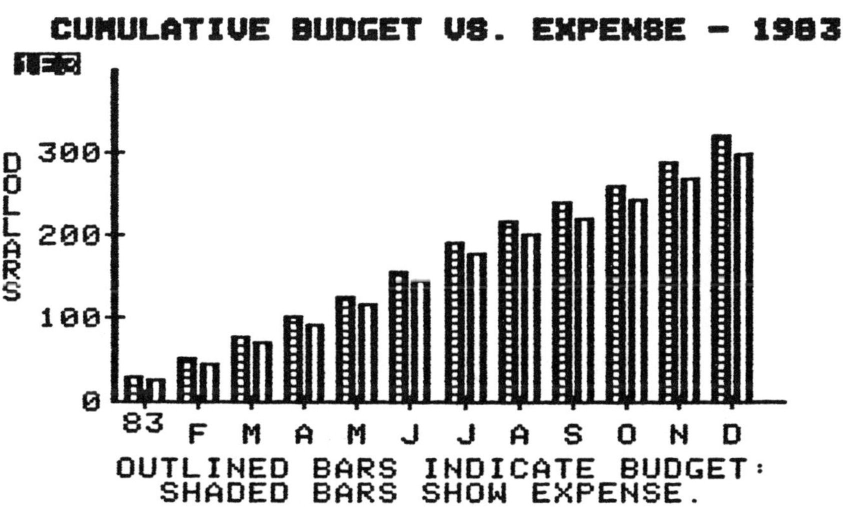

Exhibit 7-2 New Data Sets

DATE		BUDGET.T
1983	1	23456
	2	44612
	3	67506
	4	92319
	5	117818
	6	144943
	7	178395
	8	200938
	9	220160
	10	241395
	11	266382
	12	295517

DATE		EXPENSE.T
1983	1	2566
	2	5076
	3	75579
	4	100762
	5	126633
	6	154777
	7	189998
	8	214511
	9	237967
	10	259111
	11	287266
	12	318399

a table of figures showing the high and low census for a typical patient unit but with a graph produced by this set of points (Figure 7-4), it is much easier to see the trends that have developed over time. Note that although the average census has remained roughly the same, there is a smaller variation between the high and low census toward the end of the year. This fact may have implications for the way resources are allocated, because it implies that there was a time during which a low census was expected (probably the weekend) that is now a period of greater activity.

Figure 7-5 presents some additional data that have been collected and averaged on a spreadsheet program to show average daily census by day of the week for the first part of this period and the last. It shows clearly the increase in weekend activity, which would almost certainly have an effect on personnel costs resulting from the increased workload. If overtime was used to cover the vacancies, as is often the case with an unnoticed trend of this kind, the increase may be disproportionate to the revenue received.

DIETETICS

Graphics can also aid dieticians in preparing menus that are most pleasing to patients and staff in the cafeteria. By utilizing the information gathered in spreadsheets (as described in Chapter 4) or from existing

Figure 7-4 Admissions Trends: Weekly Census Graph

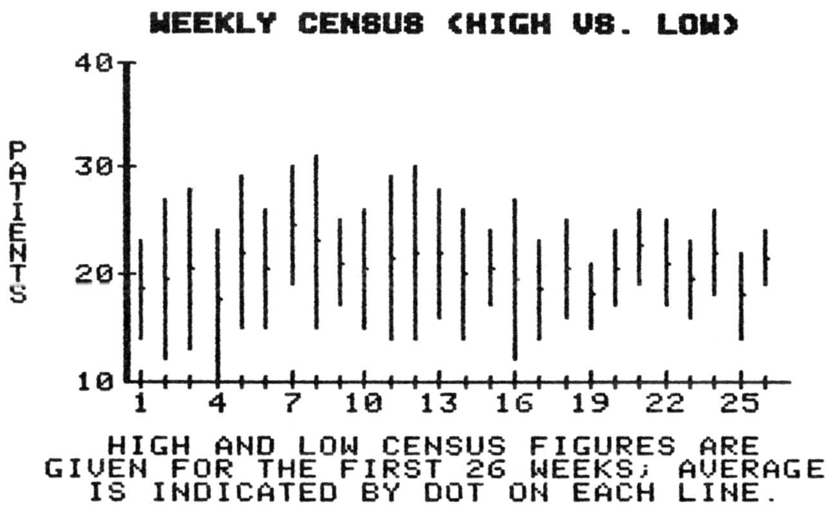

Figure 7-5 Admissions Trends: Average Daily Census Graph

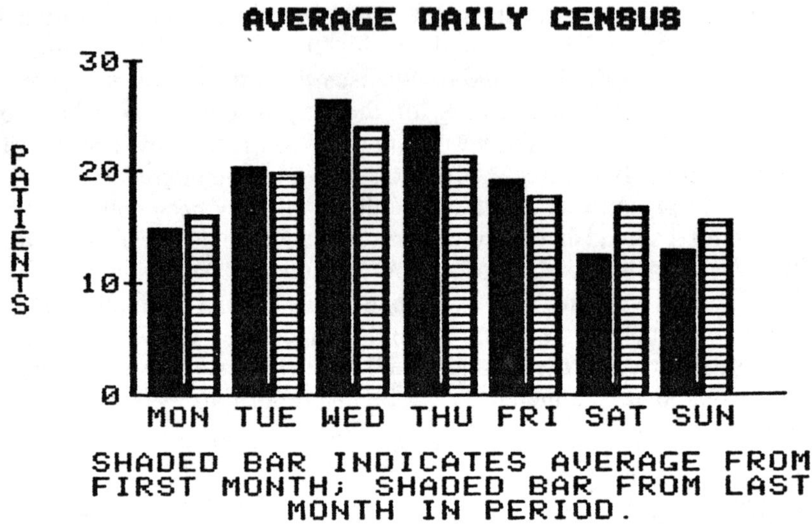

sources, graphs can be prepared showing the popularity of various items. Figure 7-6 is a pie chart showing the most popular main course during a particular month. The data were compiled using the total number of portions served during the period in question.

Figure 7-6 Menu Preparation: Pie Chart

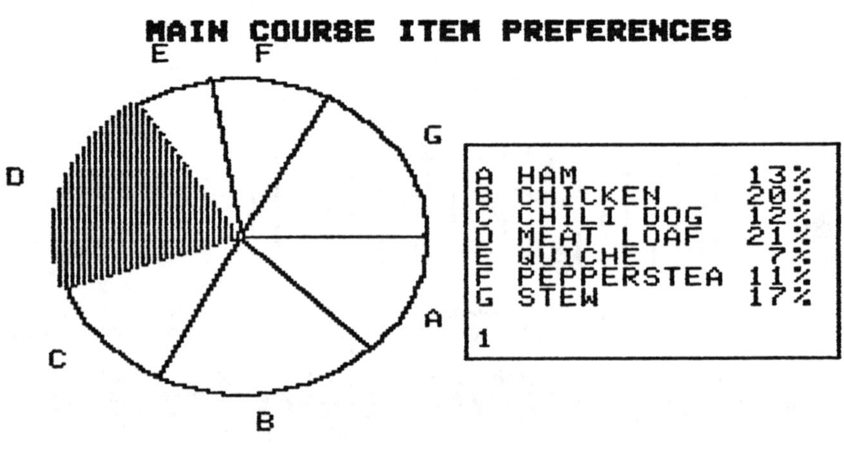

FACILITIES MANAGEMENT

An interesting way of illustrating the use of space in a health care setting is with pie charts to show the space usage by type (i.e., office, storage, utility, etc.). Exhibit 7-3 shows a typical breakdown of several kinds of space on a patient unit; in this particular example, hallway and unusable spaces are not included.

This can be compared with Figure 7-7 which shows a portion of the average distribution on all of the patient units in the institution. When administrators weigh questions regarding space usage from staff (who usually always want more), it is helpful to be able to have an easy reference regarding the unit in question. Additional information that can assist this process is found in Exhibit 7-4, which shows part of a report detailing the number of square feet of storage space divided by the number of annual patient days on that unit for each of the patient units in the facility. When performing an analysis of this nature, it is of course necessary to take into account supply needs for different types of patients (i.e., acute versus general care) to provide an accurate illustration.

Exhibit 7-3 Facilities Management: Use of Space

SPACE DISTRIBUTION

ALL UNITS

Type	Number of Spaces	Total Space	Average Per Unit	Average Room Size
Office - HN	18	1901	86	105
Office - Phys	6	740	34	123
Patient - Semi	196	44312	2014	226
Patient - Priv	85	14834	674	175
Storage - Clean	22	2450	111	111
Storage - Soild	16	876	40	55
Sunroom	6	1108	50	184

Figure 7-7 Facilities Management: Space Distribution Pie Chart

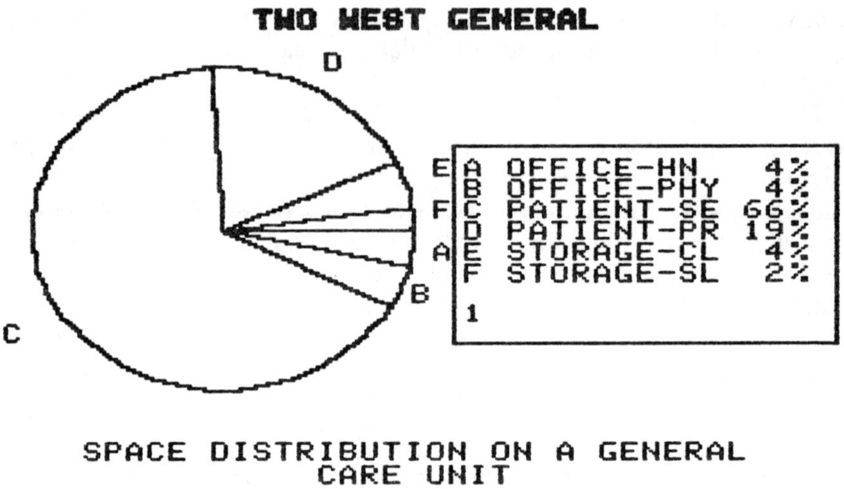

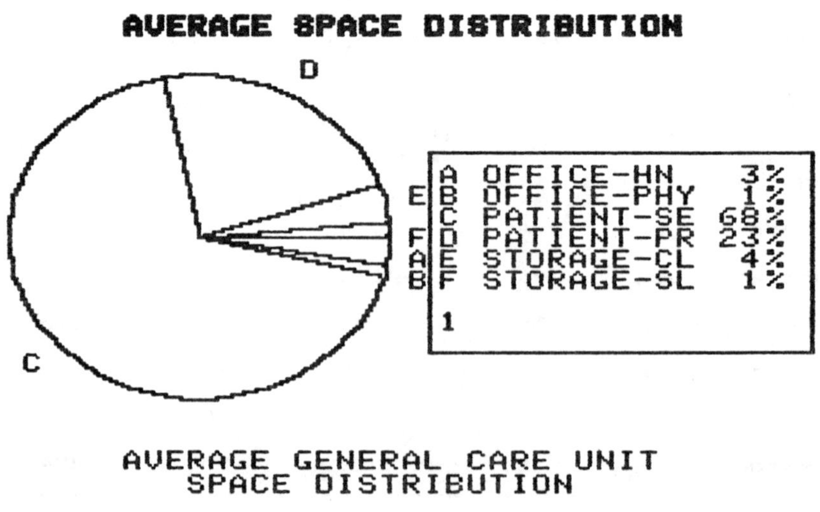

Exhibit 7-4 Facilities Management: Storage Space Analysis

SPACE DISTRIBUTION COMPARED

TO PATIENT DAYS -

ALL UNITS

Unit	Total Storage	Patient Days	Storage/ Patient Day
6 East	105	4876	.0215
6 West	98	5234	.0187
6 North	108	6109	.0177
7 West	101	5120	.0197
Surgical ICU	131	3633	.0361
Medical ICU	110	3198	.0344
7 North	125	5120	.0244

MATERIEL MANAGEMENT

Another relatively straightforward kind of analysis can be done with a graphics program that provides some additional data-manipulating routines. For example, suppose that the graphing of expense versus activity produced the graph shown in Figure 7-8. There is clearly a lag of some sort in the occurrence of the expense and the activity that produced the expense. Depending on the billing cycle at an institution, there may be a 30- to 60-day delay between the time during which an expense is incurred and the time that it is shown on a financial statement.

However, with some graphics software, a given set of data points can be "lagged" by a number of periods to produce a new set. In the example, the financial data was lagged by one month; that is, the October figure becomes the September figure, and so on. The new graph is seen in Figure 7-9, showing a much better correlation of activity with expense.

Figure 7-8 Materiel Management: Expense vs. Activity Graph

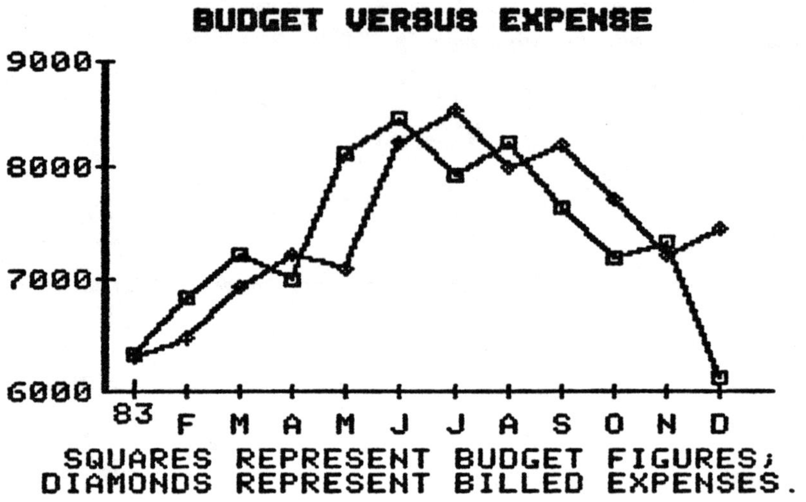

Figure 7-9 Materiel Management: Billing Graph

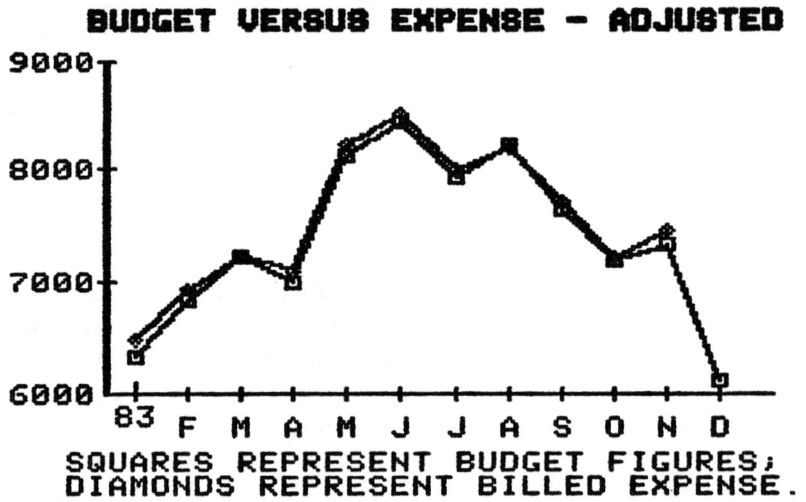

NURSING

There are a number of ways to use computer graphics to aid in projecting nurse staffing. Figure 7-10 provides a visual comparison of the three major

Figure 7-10 Staffing Projections: Nursing (Bar Graph)

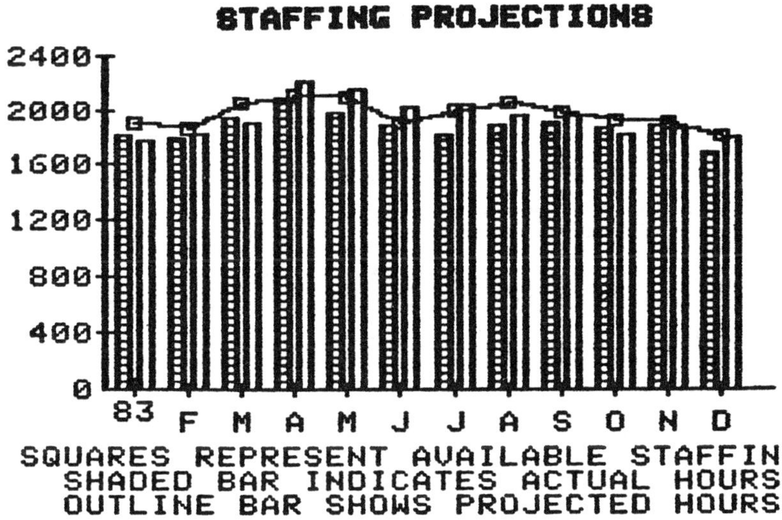
STAFFING PROJECTIONS
2400
2000
1600
1200
800
400
0
83 F M A M J J A S O N D
SQUARES REPRESENT AVAILABLE STAFFING;
SHADED BAR INDICATES ACTUAL HOURS;
OUTLINE BAR SHOWS PROJECTED HOURS.

factors discussed: the actual nurse time (R.N.) required, the projected number of hours, and the available nurse staffing.

For budgeting purposes, it can be helpful to have quantitative data on the actual time usage by staff members. Figure 7-11 shows the time utilization of a typical staff nurse; the numbers were obtained by choosing an

Figure 7-11 Staffing Projections: Nursing Time (Pie Chart)

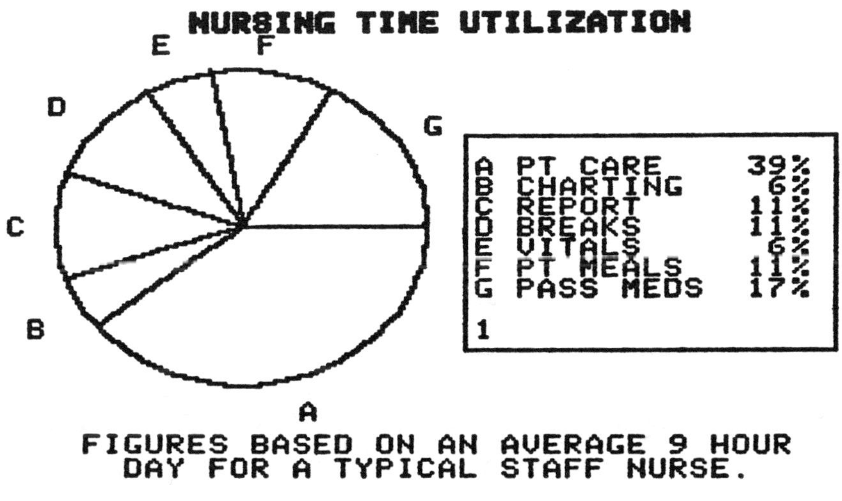

average patient load and using the time requirements previously established to find the time requirements for each task.

OPERATING ROOMS

An important issue in the financial management of an operating room suite is that of the utilization of available resources. Figure 7-12 shows this information in graphic form, comparing O.R. time available with the number of hours actually used. Note the addition of a line indicating 80 percent usage; this is provided as an aid to decision making for the future. That is, if the utilization exceeds 80 percent of the time provided on a number of occasions, a request by that department for more O.R. time might be favorably entertained.

A somewhat different approach is shown in Figure 7-13, which depicts the percent change in time usage by month. This kind of graph points out the times of the year during which utilization of staff is changing most rapidly. With this kind of information, it is possible to schedule new

---

Figure 7-12 Financial Management: O.R. Utilization Graph

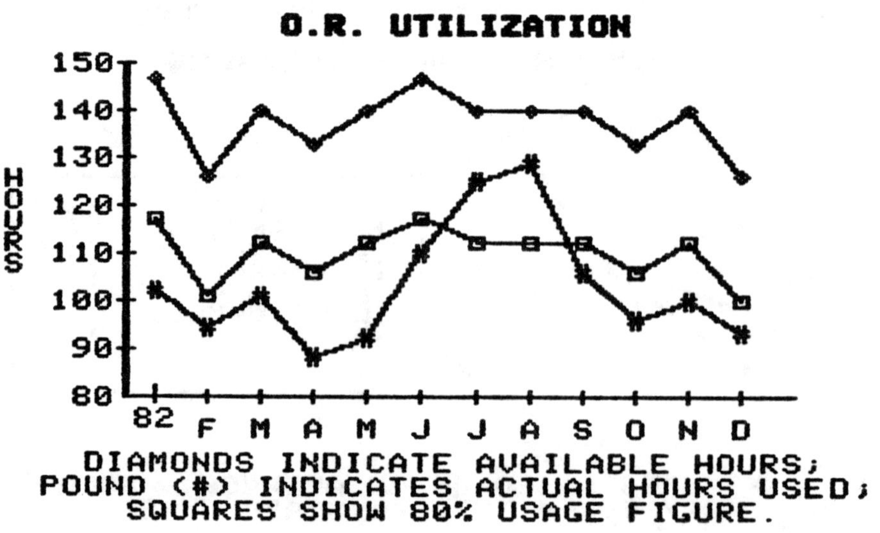

Figure 7-13 Financial Management: Time Usage Change (Bar Graph)

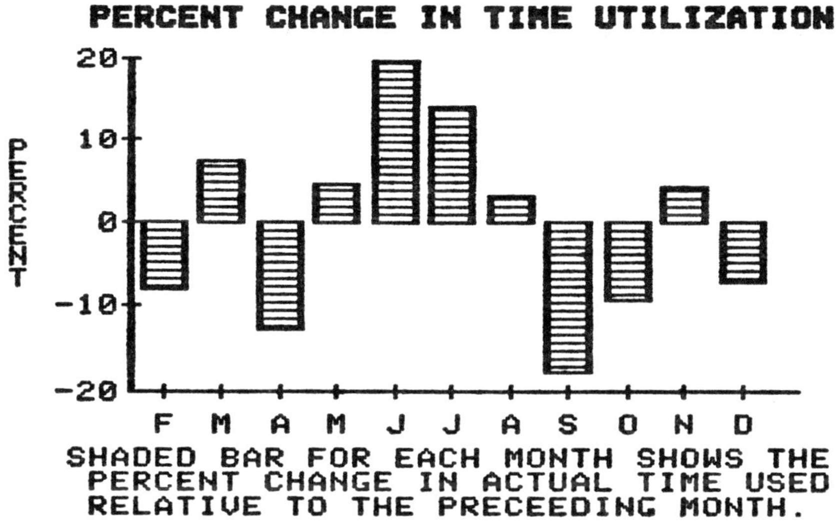

programs, training sessions, or other tasks that absorb staff time to take place during those parts of the year when "hidden" extra time should be available.

SUMMARY

As we have seen, microcomputer graphics provides an invaluable tool to the health care manager, at a very reasonable cost. The currently available software makes full use of the computer's ability to work with files of numbers, as well as pictures. Managers who are involved with the analysis of figures, both for use in personal decision making, and in providing advice to decision makers at higher organizational levels, should take the opportunity to familarize themselves with this kind of program.

Appendix A

Glossary

Arithmetic Unit—The computer component that performs arithmetic and logic operations.

Array—An arrangement of data or information elements into one or more dimensions. A two-dimensional array is called a matrix or a table.

ASCII—Abbreviation for American Standard Code of Information Interchange. Used when dealing with transfer of information from one computer to another.

BASIC—Beginners All-Purpose Symbolic Instruction Code, an easily learned high-level programming language used with many small computers.

Baud—Information transfer rate in bits per second (e.g., 1200 baud means 1200 bits per second).

Binary—The base 2 numbering system used in digital computers. Compare with the base 10 decimal system.

Bit—Binary digit. Either a zero (0) or a one (1). The lowest unit of a computer-coded word.

Boot/Bootstrap—A computer program or hardware device that brings a program into the computer from an input or storage device.

Bubble Sort—A simple method of ordering a group of items. For example, suppose you wanted to put the following list of numbers in order from greatest to smallest: 3, 7, 6, 1. The computer could be programmed to compare the first number to the second, and switch the two numbers if the second is greater than the first. In this way, the largest numbers are floated to the top of the file—hence the name "bubble" sort.

Bug—A mistake in the design of computer software or hardware that produces erroneous results.

Bus—The electrical conductor in a computer along which power or information is routed.

Busing—Transmitting or routing information or power within the computer.

Byte—Typically a group of eight bits (binary digits) that the computer operates on as a unit. Sometimes called a word.

Canned Program—See *Packaged Software.*

Cathode Ray Tube—A television-like device that allows the display of information on a screen.

Central Processing Unit—A unit of a microcomputer that includes the circuits controlling the interpretation and execution of instructions.

Coaxial Cable—A special form of wiring used to connect one computer with another that provides two data paths to allow for simultaneous communication in both directions.

CPU—See *Central Processing Unit.*

CRT—See *Cathode Ray Tube.*

Cursor—The point on the screen at which the user may enter text. It is typically indicated with a flashing box or line.

Custom Software—Programs written for a specific job or purpose.

Daisy Wheel Printer—A printer that uses a daisy wheel shaped print element; i.e., the letters are placed on the surface of the ends of the "spokes" of a "wheel."

Data—The most elemental units of factual material used as a basis for processing, decision, or discussion. The term denotes aggregated letters, numbers, or other symbols and represents the most basic information that can be processed by a computer.

Data Base—The term used to describe all of the information available to a computer program.

Data Base Management (DBM)—A process by which information is stored and retrieved so that it may be used.

Data Base Management Program—A program that processes (sort, collate, merge) data from a data base to produce or maintain a specific information set.

Data Processing (DP)—Generic term usually signifying the electronic processing of data and information using computers.

Debug—To identify and correct errors in computer software and hardware.

Dedicated—Exclusively assigned to a specific task; said of a piece of computer hardware or software.

Disk—An input/output device in the form of a flat platter resembling a phonograph record. Disk surfaces consist of a magnetic recording medium for electronic storage of data. Disks may be hard or flexible (floppy). Hard disks are capable of storing much more data than floppy disks.

Disk Drive—A mechanical device that provides for the storage of computer programs and data on diskettes coated with special magnetic media (see Chapter 2).

Disk Operating System (DOS)—A software program that allows the user to make use of a disk drive.

DOS—See *Disk Operating System.*

Dot-Matrix Printer—A printer that forms letters and other characters to convey information by using an array of pins that strike a ribbon against the paper or by spraying jets of ink dots to achieve a similar printing result. See also *Ink Jet Printer.*

Download—To take data from another computer system into one's own computer. For example, a manager may wish to obtain a large amount of detailed information relating to activity in his area that is present in a mainframe computer system, and use it as the basis for a series of reports. It is obviously preferable to get the data in machine-readable form, rather than type it back in from paper records. The manager would have to convince the data processing manager to "download," that is, send the data from the mainframe to the microcomputer (usually over a phone line).

DP—See *Data Processing.*

EDP—See *Electronic Data Processing.*

Electronic Data Processing (EDP)—Usually abbreviated to Data Processing. See *Data Processing.*

Electronic Spreadsheet—A program that allows the user to develop tabular information similar to that on an accountant's columnar pad. Information in the rows and columns can be manipulated electronically, through the use of replicable formats, calculations, and algorithms. Electronic spreadsheets are designed to save time by eliminating the drudgery of repetitive calculations, corrections, and typing.

Field—A portion of a computer record that contains one data item. For example, if a personnel file containing a record for each employee were kept, each record might include the employee's name, address, home phone, and social security number. Each of these individual facts would occupy a field in the record.

File—A number of records grouped in some way under a common heading.

Filename—The name that the user gives to a file of data stored by a computer.

Firmware—A term denoting programs permanently residing in a computer's Read Only Memory (ROM). Compare with *Software* and *Hardware*.

Floppy Disk—See *Disk*.

Flowchart—A block-type diagram that provides graphic representation of a computer program.

FORTRAN—FORmula TRANslation, a high-level scientific programming language usually used with large computers.

Graphics—A capability designed into some computers allowing them to present information in a pictorial format (e.g., pie charts or bar graphs), rather than mere alphanumeric characters.

Graphics Interface Card—A special printer interface card that allows the printing of graphic images by a dot-matrix printer. The card itself is a circuit board that plugs into the computer, forming a communications link between the computer and the printer.

Hard Copy—Computer output printed on paper.

Hard Disk—See *Disk*.

Hardware—The computer's physical parts. See also *Firmware, Software*.

Hardwired—Several computer systems that are connected by permanently installed coaxial cable, rather than by a temporary phone link. In general, it represents a permanent physical solution versus a more flexible approach to a problem.

IC—See *Integrated Circuit*.

Ink Jet Printer—See *Dot-Matrix Printer*.

Input—Data to be entered or being entered into a computer. This term also describes the act of entering data.

Input/Output—This term may refer either to data or to an I/O device such as a printer, keyboard, or disk drive.

Input Unit—A device used for entering data into a computer, such as a keyboard or disk drive.

Integrated Circuit (IC)—Interconnected elements forming a microcircuit etched on a single crystal or semiconductor.

Interface—Equipment that allows two computer units to operate jointly (such as a keyboard and CPU).

Interface Card—A hardware device inserted into a slot within the computer to allow it to communicate via cable with another hardware device, e.g., a printer.

I/O—See *Input/Output*.

Joystick—A pointing device used to maneuver the cursor on the screen.

K—Abbreviation for "Kilo," meaning "thousand." Computer memory is often specified in terms of thousands of bytes. The main memory of 64K or 64K bytes means a memory capacity of 64,000 bytes.

Keyboard—A set of alphanumeric and other symbolic characters arranged on keys in a manner resembling a typewriter. Pressing a key causes the character to be entered into the computer.

Kludge—A slang term for a quick (and probably inadequate) repair of a program error.

Large Scale Integration (LSI)—The placement of a large number of circuits on a single chip (typically 1,000 or more).

LCD (Liquid Crystal Diode)—A special display using a flat panel to show data. It has the advantage of taking up much less space than a cathode ray tube, which uses a projection method.

Letter-Quality Printer—A printer that utilizes fully formed characters (like an ordinary typewriter) in printing. Compare with *Dot-Matrix Printer.*

Liquid Crystal Diode—See *LCD.*

Load—To enter data and/or instructions into the computer, often from a disk or tape drive.

Logic—A term used to designate the part of the computer that makes logical decisions, such as A is equal to B, or X is greater than Y.

LSI—See *Large Scale Integration.*

Mainframe—A synonym for CPU. Most popularly, a synonym used to denote large computer CPUs.

Mega—Prefix for "million." One Megabyte equals a million bytes.

Memory/Main Memory—The computer's internal memory, as opposed to its peripheral or external memory (disks, tapes).

Menu—A list of the programs or program steps that are available to the user.

Micro—Prefix for "millionth." Microcomputers are sometimes called "micros." The prefix denotes something very small.

Microcomputer—A term used to designate a small computer, often a personal computer but also a small professional computer designed for professional rather than casual or home use.

Microprocessor—The central processing unit (CPU) of a microcomputer.

Minicomputer—A small, intermediate computer, sized between the microcomputer and the large computer. Minicomputers are often differentiated from microcomputers in that they are often multiple- rather than single-user machines. Minicomputers usually require much larger amounts of space; the CPU, unlike that of the microcomputer, is usually free standing, rather than table top in design.

Modem—Modulator/Demodulator, a device for sending and receiving information, usually over the telephone.

Mouse—A pointing device used with some microcomputers.

Output—The data or information coming out of a computer in any form, such as on a CRT, printer, etc.

Output Unit—A device (CRT, printer) for handling the data or information coming out of a computer.

Packaged Software—Generic programs that can be purchased and that are designed to perform a specific purpose such as data base management or word processing. These programs require user adaptation rather than being adapted to the user. Often called *Canned Software*.

Peripheral—A piece of equipment that operates in conjunction with a computer, such as a printer or CRT.

Personal Computer—A small microcomputer that usually provides modest data processing capabilities for individual, often casual, users.

Pixel—The smallest single point of light on the computer screen that is fully controllable by the computer, and provides a measure of the resolution provided by the computer in graphic displays.

Printer—A computer output device that produces printed copy.

Processor—The central processing unit (CPU) of the computer.

Program/Programmer—A set of written instructions in a language or code that can be used by a computer. The programmer is the person who writes the instructions.

RAM—See *Random Access Memory*.

Random Access Memory (RAM)—The internal "scratchpad" or space used by the computer to store instructions and data; formed by integrated circuits within the computer.

Read—What a computer does when it accesses data from a computer disk, tape, or other input device or medium in order to process or store it.

Read Only Memory (ROM)—Internal computer memory that can be "read" by the computer but not changed. ROM contains the permanent instructions used by the computer to perform various tasks such as screen formatting, keyboard control, and logical functions.

Record—A group of data elements that are collected together to provide information about a person, place, thing, or event.

ROM—See *Read Only Memory*.

Soft Copy—Information displayed on a CRT rather than in printed form. See *Hard Copy.*

Software—Computer programs. See *Program/Programmer.* See also *Hardware, Firmware.*

Spooling—Temporary storage of data to be printed, allowing the computer to process other information while also directing the printer. Because the computer divides its attention, performance speed of each task is degraded.

Turnkey—A computer system that can be installed and used with no additional programming effort by the user. The user simply turns the key and it runs.

Utility—A program that is part of the operating system of the computer and that performs a specific task, such as a sort routine.

Word Processing (WP)—A computer program that allows letters, words, phrases, sentences, and larger groupings of characters to be entered, edited, displayed, and printed.

WP—See *Word Processing.*

Wraparound—The capability of a word processing program to automatically start a new line on the computer display without breaking any words, and without the user pressing the RETURN key.

Write—What a computer does when it places or sends data to a disk, tape, or other memory device for storage or processing.

Appendix B

How To Design, Write, and Implement a Microcomputer Program from Scratch

Computer programming can be both rewarding and enjoyable; setting up your own program can make the maximum use of a microcomputer's potential and enhance your own creativity and productivity. The material that follows is in no way a complete primer for software development—there are numerous textbooks available on this subject—but it can serve as an introduction and guide that will ease the process.

DEFINE PURPOSE AND NECESSARY INPUT

You will want to carefully define the purpose of your program as well as the input required. Check the cost of gathering the needed data and the availability of the data (it may be restricted or the "property" of someone else in the organization). It is also a good idea to determine who will use the program. In general, it is best to program for the person who is totally lacking in computer expertise.

DETERMINE WHAT NEEDS TO BE DONE

The first step in examining the problem is to consider the size of the task to be accomplished (see Appendix C). If you would like to write (or have written) a custom program for a microcomputer, the best place to start is with existing systems, if any. There are several reasons for this:

1. The data gathering techniques used can be kept, with some modification. If your aim is to expand an existing report, you can get some idea of the increased cost in gathering additional data.

2. The data gathered are probably what you will continue using. The volume of data will help you decide whether you need a floppy disk drive or a hard disk for storage.
3. The process of producing the report will demonstrate the necessary algorithms for translating the raw data into the finished report.
4. The finished report gives you a place to start with your own output format.

DETERMINE NECESSARY ALGORITHMS

The next step is to determine the algorithms needed for the program. Since most management reports tend to use a few formulas for a large amount of data, this is typically the easiest part of the task.

DEFINE OUTPUT

Definition of the output is an important step. Check with those who are to receive the report to see if it meets the need for which it is intended.

DECIDE ON PROGRAM LANGUAGE

Most computers come equipped with some form of BASIC; although denigrated by computer purists, BASIC is not a bad language for programming. However, other languages should also be considered, for several reasons. First, BASIC is an interpreted language; this means that each statement in the program is translated into machine language every time it is read. A compiled language goes through the program once, translates the whole program into machine language, and then runs this version; this results in a program that runs from two to ten times faster.

If your program contains a good deal of numerical computation or manipulation of text, you should seriously consider using a compiled language, such as Pascal. Although there are compilers available for BASIC, many of them have inconvenient restrictions when used with microcomputers, particularly with those having only 64K of memory.

GETTING DOWN TO WRITING

Having completed a first pass through the design phase, go back and check your assumptions. This is particularly important if you are doing this task along with many others and several months have elapsed.

In writing the program, it is a good idea to break it up into the following areas:

1. Outer shell
2. Data entry and output
3. Necessary algorithms
4. File storage and record retrieval and modification

The outer shell segment is the portion that controls the flow of work in the program. For example, the Facilities Space Inventory program uses an outer shell that consists mostly of the main menu, a few routines, and directions on what files to call up for the rest of the program functions. If the View/Alter option is chosen, the corresponding file on the diskette is activated and placed in the machine, overwriting the original outer shell segment. When you are done with View/Alter, the outer shell is reloaded from the diskette, overwriting the View/Alter section program. Dividing a program into a number of smaller subprograms is a common technique in microcomputer programming because of the relatively small internal memory spaces involved.

The data entry routines should be suited to the user. They should be designed for convenience, matching the manner in which the data are collected. There should also be some attempt to catch human errors in the form of poor typing and incorrectly formatted inputs; this becomes very important if anyone but the programmer is to use the program. The output and algorithms should already have been checked and defined as above.

File storage and retrieval will constitute the main portion of the program. It is this section that allows the user to store the data needed from one work session to another and to view and modify this data if needed. In most applications, random access files are best. As you may recall from Chapter 6, every record is of a certain declared size, which allows the computer to find a given record easily. Although there is some wasted space with this file type, the increase in speed is most desirable.

PROGRAMMING POINTERS

Write out, and check over, the entire program before entering one line of code in the computer. The temptation is to sit down and start typing away; this can result in much time spent trying to fix something that should not have been entered in the first place.

Be sure to document completely as you write. You will find that program steps written the week before become meaningless hieroglyphics without adequate documentation, particularly when programming in BASIC. The choice of language can be very important here; Pascal is an ideal language in this sense, because it allows the use of long variable names. For example, it is easier to remember the purpose of a variable named MonthlyBudget(X) than one called MB(X).

During the writing process, it is a good idea to review your objectives once again; make sure that all of your assumptions still hold true.

After the program is running, go through and carefully check all output for mathematical and text accuracy. Do a complete runthrough by hand to make sure that the system is working properly.

Also, it is important to try to test as much of the system as possible. This includes testing every option, every algorithm, under a number of different conditions. Type nonsense into the program every now and then to test error checking. Fill up a disk with data. Ask for the impossible and see if the program can handle it. Ideally, the programmer should do to the program exactly what other users will do; they will make data entry errors, they will overfill diskettes, they will try to delete files to be saved, and, in general, they will abuse the program.

There are three distinct periods in which bugs tend to appear in programs. The first is, of course, when the programmer develops the output of the program (as well as the other routines, such as input and file storage). The second occurs when the other users of the program figure out methods of input, switching of diskettes, and other activities undreamed of by the program author. If the error checking routines are inadequate, these will result in the dread epiphany of strange and obscure bugs in the program. They were there all the time, of course; it just takes the appropriate sequence of events to make them come to light.

The third period in which errors appear is after a relative lull in which the programmer fools himself or herself into believing that all of the bugs have been found. During this period, the users are filling the diskettes with data and stretching the program to its limits. Depending on the degree to which the program was tested by the author, a whole new crop of bugs related to this new level of user sophistication will appear.

GOING PUBLIC

Having written and tested the program, the next step is to introduce it to the people who will be using it. Make sure that they understand all parts of the program, how to take care of the machine and the program diskettes, and how to make backup copies of data entered. Information contained in Chapter 3 should be particularly helpful.

The last step is to circulate the finished report—and enjoy the applause.

Appendix C

Calculating the Size of the Task

In order to determine the best manner in which to proceed in solving a problem with computer assistance, it is necessary to consider the size of the task to be accomplished. The terms and concepts needed for this process are contained in Chapter 2 and should be reviewed before proceeding. Appendix B contains a brief set of instructions from a systems point of view.

The first step is to break the task down into three parts, as follows:

1. Data required, and the form in which it will be entered
2. The finished product defined (format and content)
3. Algorithms that lead from step 1 to step 2

The data required by the program will be a combination of the following types:

1. Numerical (e.g., a budget figure such as $347.45)
2. Text strings (e.g., a string of characters such as Monthly Report)

It is also necessary to include all of the data required to produce the report, not just the particular numbers that will appear in the printed text, if the computer is to perform the necessary calculation. For example, a summary report might fit all on one page and contain perhaps 100 numbers; the report itself, however, may be based on thousands of figures.

The manner of data entry is important, because the programmer must make a choice between providing a manner convenient to the user and a manner convenient to the machine. This is a particularly important point if you are trying to make use of canned software, which typically offers only one data entry format. An example of the problems encountered is that of a program requiring the random entry of diverse forms of data which must be presented in an ordered way in a final report. The spreadsheet programs, for example, do not provide convenient sort capabilities.

Also, some canned software programs require a certain amount of expertise on the part of even the casual user. A simple task like entering the figures from the most recent month for a report may take an expert user. By comparison, a specially written program may provide a data entry format usable by anyone available, even those with virtually no computer experience.

The algorithms that produce the final figures from the raw data involved are important because they may limit the kind of program that can be used. For example, some canned software programs will allow only very limited forms of calculation or sorting, whereas others will allow the entry of complex, specialized formulas.

When considering the amount of data required, it is important to determine the following:

1. How much of the data is to be kept from one sitting to the next time the program is used
2. How much of the data has to fit in the machine at a time while the report is being prepared

The problem can be broadly stated as being one of data storage. As we have seen in the preceding chapters, the RAM (or internal) memory of the machine is typically at a premium in microcomputers. Most micros are limited to 64-128K bytes of storage; of this amount, about 30,000 bytes are taken up by the program and other operating systems vital to the computer. The following illustrates the use of memory by a typical software program:

Number of bytes available	64,000
Bytes required for BASIC language	−16,000
Bytes required for Disk Operating System (DOS)	−10,000
Bytes required for program	−14,000
Bytes remaining for data	24,000

If you are thinking of purchasing a computer system, the amount of data storage available with a given combination of hardware and software is a particularly important consideration. In the preceding example, the user should question the amount of data storage available in the machine. Does this represent a limit to the size of the data file that may be used? In the case of a program such as AppleWriter, a word processing program, the data storage in the machine represents a limit to the size of the text file that may be manipulated. However, in programs that are disk-based (using the disk drive storage to keep portions of a file manipulated), the size of the internal RAM used is relatively unimportant; instead, the user should be concerned with the amount of space available on a diskette.

The basic principle is to minimize the time and effort to produce a usable final report; the manner in which the report is produced (the "elegance" of the method) is unimportant. This can be accomplished by using the following guidelines for problem solving with micros:

1. Use the spreadsheet programs if possible. The ease of setting up the program and the basically simple, intuitively obvious data entry makes it the clear choice for a first try. It is much easier to modify a spreadsheet than to modify most data base management programs. Custom-written software is typically the most difficult to modify. Remember that a 64K micro has about 32K of space for data in a spreadsheet, 94K in a 128K machine, and about 180K in a 256K machine.
2. If your data requirements are somewhat larger (storage of up to a million bytes per year for a particular application), try the data base management programs. Although they are more difficult to work with and have limited report generation capability, you will still save effort with such programs.
3. If your data requirements exceed a million bytes per application, and you have special requirements with regard to input or output formats, you will almost certainly have to go with a larger mass storage device than a floppy disk. When using hard disk drives, remember that not all canned software devices can easily access these drives.
4. If the application is one involving a DBM effort over several years, in a well-established format, it will probably repay your efforts to develop a custom-written program.

Index

I

J

K

L

M

N

O

P

R

S

About the Authors

William W. Christensen is the Administrative Associate of the W.K. Kellogg Eye Center of the University of Michigan Hospitals. He has a strong background in health care management and the management uses of the microcomputer in the health care environment. He was an honors student at the University of Michigan and has worked in hospitals since 1973. Mr. Christensen has used microcomputers in financial, facility, and environmental management since 1979, and has written sophisticated data base programs relating to these activities. In addition, he teaches courses in introductory microcomputing and financial management and also does consulting to large organizations in the use of microcomputer systems.

Eugene I. Stearns has been Associate Administrator of the Main Hospital and the W.K. Kellogg Eye Center of the University of Michigan Hospitals since 1979. He began his health care management career in 1968 as director of medical information in a large teaching hospital. Mr. Stearns holds a masters degree in library science from Kent State University with a concentration in automated information retrieval systems. With Mr. Christensen, he has co-authored several articles and they have also collaborated on a series of seminars. In addition, he consults in the area of medical information systems.